ESSENTIAL OILS FROM THE GROUND UP

A Materials Science Professor looks at the Phenomenon of Young Living

J. A. von Fraunhofer

MSc, PhD, FADM, FASM, FRSC

Professor Emeritus

University of Maryland, Baltimore

Essential oils from the Ground Up by J. A. von Fraunhofer

ISBN 978-1-952027-98-7 (Paperback)
ISBN 978-1-952027-99-4 (Hardback)

Printed in the United States of America.

New Leaf Media, LLC
175 S. 3rd Street, Suite 200
Columbus, OH 43215
www.thenewleafmedia.com

Dedication

To Susan, the light of my life and whose
love, support and encouragement
make all the difference.

Acknowledgement

The author should like to thank his good friend Dr. R. Michael Buch for all his sage advice and helpful comments during the writing of this book.

In Memoriam

The year, 2019, marked the 25th anniversary of the founding of Young Living by D. Gary Young. This celebration, however, was marred by the sad loss of Gary Young in 2018. He leaves a wife, Mary, and his two children but also an incredible legacy.

Gary Young is rightfully known as the "father" of the modern essential oil industry in the United States and, possibly, Internationally. His approach to growing essential oil source plants, their harvesting and processing transformed essential oils from a "cottage industry" into a technologically based, highly efficient and very successful corporation that supplies essential oils and essential oil-based products to a worldwide market. His processing innovations, essential oil formulations and meticulous attention to product quality and purity together with growing plants on Young Living's own farms using ecologically sound principles have made the Young Living company and its products the standard for the industry.

Although Gary Young will be missed by all members of the Young Living family and members, his legacy will live on in the quality and purity of products and the dedication to service that characterized him personally and the company he founded a quarter of a century ago. We should all be grateful to Gary Young for what he achieved and promoted with essential oils and the incredible benefits that his pioneering efforts have accomplished throughout the world. Gary Young's legacy will be proudly maintained by the company and its worldwide membership.

Contents

FOREWORD

Scientific inquiry starts with one word…**why**? For example, why does water freeze at 0°C (32°F) and boil at 100°C (212°F)? What is the structure of water and why can it be poured? The drive to answer seemingly simple questions impels science and scientists forward. This book was written because I wondered why the small bottles of Young Living essential oils cost more than bottles of ostensibly the same oil that can be purchased in chain stores across the country. We all know that name brands always cost more than "no name" products and name-brand pharmaceuticals cost more, often considerably so, than generic drugs. So why is there a price differential for essential oils?

Obviously, there is more at play here than simply good marketing but what is it and is the difference between products that great? This book is the result of careful inquiry into these questions. As one successful company claims…better ingredients make better pizzas. What are the "better ingredients" of Young Living essential oils?

I became interested in essential oils by accident. When I was an undergraduate studying chemistry at the then Sir John Cass College, University of London, there were lectures on all aspects of chemistry and that included terpenes and terpenoids, the principal components of essential oils. Once I graduated and went into the "real world" of R&D, much of the information that I had so diligently acquired was relegated to the dim, dark and cobwebbed recesses of my mind. That was the situation for decades until serendipity stepped in.

A good friend of mine and outstanding scientist surprised me by moving from Big Pharma into a senior position within the essential oil industry, vaguely re-awakening my interest in terpenes. Not too much later I read an article entitled *Smarter smells. After years of research, the flavor and fragrance industry is increasingly turning to biotechnology for commercial production.* This article brought home to me the fact that I had simply forgotten, or perhaps never knew much about the complex organic molecules essential to the flavor and fragrance industry. It was immediately obvious to my cynical mind that the cost and scarcity of essential oils was an open invitation for disreputable companies to generate big profits by incorporating synthetic ingredients into what should be wholly natural products. It also became obvious that the complex mixtures of chemicals known as essential oils that are derived from plants are very important in economic, biological and pharmacological terms but they are a largely neglected area in mainstream chemistry. Even standard organic chemistry textbooks barely mention them.

So, now that my interest was thoroughly awakened, I started to think about the complex subjects of flavors and fragrances. I have previously written a short monograph entitled *Vitamins, Minerals and Spices* in which I discussed how important spices are to human health and gastronomy, but I didn't delve into essential oils *per se.* Nevertheless, it is obvious that the essential oils in spices are drawn out by cooking to provide the flavors and delicious smells of food. Not only that, the incredibly appealing scents of flowers and plants are wholly due to the essential oils within those plants.

Given the evocative effects of essential oils liberated from botanicals, it is unsurprising that there is a major, and growing, interest in the mental and physical health benefits of aromatherapy. In fact, companies such as Young Living market essential oils and diffusers that provide this important therapy. In addition to aromatherapy, there are growing numbers of products based on essential oils that provide numerous overall health, skin and other benefits for their users. Clearly, essential oils are BIG business, and their associated physical and mental health benefits are remarkable.

This raises the question of what is involved in extracting an essential oil from a plant to provide a bottle of oil, a bar of soap or a jar of cream? Just thinking about this was the stimulus to get started on this book because I wanted to know what Young Living's "Seed to Seal" corporate logo actually involved.

This book provides a guide to the phenomenon of Young Living and its essential oils by discussing what essential oils are, where they come from and how they are extracted. It also considers the many analytical and quality control procedures of the company as well as the infrastructure that takes essential oils from seeds in the ground to the diversity of products for which the company is famous. This book also indicates the extra-ordinary scope of essential oils in treating an incredibly wide variety of conditions that can affect the health and happiness of the human body.

J. A. von Fraunhofer

CHAPTER 1

INTRODUCTION

To the average person, essential oils are slightly oily liquids that come in small bottles and are, by and large, quite expensive. On the other hand, these small bottles last a long time and can have remarkable effects on the body and mind. These simple statements cover a whole lot of information but to understand them and their importance, it is necessary to dig a little more deeply into what essentials oils are, where they come from, how they are obtained and what makes them so special.

Basically, an essential oil is a concentrated hydrophobic (water-repelling) liquid containing volatile aroma compounds that are extracted from plants (botanicals). Essential oils are also known as volatile oils, ethereal oils or, more simply, as the oil of the plant from which it is extracted. These oils are "essential" in that they contain the "essence" of the plant's aroma, that is, the characteristic fragrance of the plants from which they were extracted. Essential oils are used in perfumes, cosmetics, soap, domestic products and in food flavoring. They are also burned as incense, diluted with a carrier oil and applied in massage therapy as well as diffused in air with a nebulizer (vaporizer or diffuser) for aromatherapy.

Commercially, essential oils are generally extracted by distillation, often combined with the injection of steam into the still or distillation vessel to help release the oil from the plant, as discussed in Chapter 3.

Historical Perspective

Now, having set the scene, it might be interesting to consider the history of essential oils because they have been around almost since the dawn of civilization. The early methods used for extracting essential oils and when (and how) they were first used is lost in the mists of antiquity but essential oil extraction by distillation has been practiced for thousands of years. In fact, distillation was practiced at around the same time that hieroglyphic writing was developed along with the establishment of the Sumerian civilization, the invention of the chariot and the founding of Egypt's First Dynasty. Incidentally, the oldest known medical treatise was also written during this time period. So, not only has man been distilling alcoholic beverages and likely extracting essential oils by distillation for some 5000 years but treating different ailments with various medications and drinking alcohol have been important since the earliest of times.

The earliest recorded mention of the techniques and methods used to produce essential oils is believed to be that of the Andalusian botanist, pharmacist, physician and scientist Ibn al-Baitar or Ibn al-Baytar (1197–1248 AD[1]). Interestingly, the name al-Baitar means *son of the veterinarian* and suggests that even back in the 12th Century, veterinary science was well-established within the Islamic culture. This is in sharp contrast to the intolerance towards science and Hippocratic medicine, and even bathing, exhibited throughout Europe in the Dark Ages.

Although it is unknown when essential oils were first used in cosmetics and perfumes as well as for medicinal purposes, it appears that Ibn al-Baitar was the first to systematically record the contributions to medical science made by Islamic physicians during the Middle Ages. These physicians added some 300-400 different types of medicine to the 1000 or more in use since antiquity. Further, al-Baitar in the 13th Century compiled the *Compendium on Simple Medicaments and Foods* which was a pharmacopoeia (or pharmaceutical encyclopedia) that listed 1400 plants, foods, and drugs, and their medicinal uses. This treatise was organized alphabetically by the name of the medici-

---

1   In this book, the abbreviations BC and AD are used for dating historical events. These abbreviations correspond to the recently developed usages of BCE ("Before the Common Era") and CE ("Common Era.").

nal plant, plant component or other substance and, interestingly, the vast majority of medications covered were botanicals. What is also significant is that al-Baitar cited the earlier written works of some 150 Arabic and 20 Greek physicians. Further, this book was translated and published in both French and German as late as the 19th Century. Ibn al-Baitar also provided detailed chemical information on the production of rosewater and orange water and discussed the extraction of essential oils from flowers and leaves by hot oils and fats, that is, hot enfleurage. Apparently, the oils used for this purpose were expressed from olives and sesame seeds. Further, al-Baitar wrote that essential oils also were extracted by distillation and indicated that the distillation product comprised condensed water containing scented droplets which were used as perfume and for producing the costliest medications.

The subject of extracting essential oils from their parent botanicals is addressed in greater detail in Chapter 3 but central to this issue is the importance of the quality of the parent plants. Although not explicitly stated, the important factors determining the quality of all plants and trees used as sources of essential oils include where they are grown. Consequently, the local climate conditions, the mineral and salts in the ground water, whether they have been exposed to artificial fertilizers and herbicides and even the quality and mineral content of the earth in which they grow are all influence the quality of the sources of essential oils. These horticultural principles are well-known to gardeners and agronomists the world over.

Consumers can recognize the difference, for example, between olive oil from Italy, Spain, Greece and Turkey. Likewise, most wine lovers can readily distinguish between varietal wines[2] produced from grapes gathered in different countries, different locations within the same country and even within the same State. Some oenophiles go so far as to claim to be able to distinguish between wines made from grapes grown on different sides of the same valley. The year in which the grapes were grown can also markedly the quality (and price!) of a wine and this marked effect on "vintage" clearly indicates the importance of climactic and other conditions during that year's growth cycle.

---

2   Varietal wines are those made primarily from a single named grape variety.

There is, in fact, a term *terroir*[3] that is intended to encompass all the various environmental, horticultural, geographical and even cultural influences that impact the growing of grapes, their harvesting and the process of wine making. The same term should also be applied to essential oils because of the myriad influences that affect them and their properties.

It follows, therefore, that the properties and characteristics of nominally the same essential oil from a named plant source will be modified, and often markedly influenced, in such characteristics as aroma and health benefits by the growth factors outlined above. This is an important principle in the production of essential oils. When extracted oils from different source materials are compounded or mixed together, the resultant essential oil can often be unsatisfactory. It is the careful adherence to the cultivation of plant materials that distinguishes Young Living essential oils from those of many competitors and, particularly, cheaper products that are claimed to 100% pure. Young Living has well-controlled and carefully monitored orchards and plant farms all over the world to ensure the highest quality of their products.

Finally, it is important to introduce the word *organic* when discussing agricultural products and food. As readers will note, organic compounds have already been mentioned in the Foreword and in this chapter, but this term was never really explained. In fact, the word *organic* has two meanings/applications in science. The first is in *Organic Chemistry*, a major subdiscipline in chemistry and encompasses the scientific study of the structure, properties and reactions of the various forms of matter that contain carbon atoms. In other words, this is the field of chemistry dealing with what are known as organic compounds and organic materials.

More commonly in modern parlance, the term *organic* refers to foods farmed using practices that promote balance and biodiversity throughout the environment. Thus, "organic" foods and botanicals are grown without the use of pesticides, herbicides and artificial fertilizers. Further, organic foods should not have been treated with or contain synthetic food additives and have not been exposed to solvents or irradiation other than natural sunlight. Organic farming of

---

3   *Terroir* is a French word derived from the Latin *terra* or *territorium* denoting "a stretch of land limited by its agricultural capacity."

animals and poultry adheres to the same restrictions when they were raised, and the term indicates that they were not treated with antibiotics or exposed to radiation or pesticides in their food. The limitations imposed by claims of organic farming are important because, unfortunately, agrochemicals, notably pesticides, are dangerous and they are responsible for about 200,000 deaths every year with most of these fatalities occurring in developing countries.[4] Consequently, scientific advisers have suggested to the UN Human Rights Council that pesticide use is endangering basic human rights to nutritional food and overall health. Further, there is increasing evidence that certain herbicides and weed killers are wreaking havoc on bee populations worldwide. Consequently, responsible producers of essential oils like Young Living insist on carefully controlled farming of the plants grown to make their products.

4   Maria Burke. Pesticide use 'threatens human rights', UN advisers claim. Chemistry World (2017) 14(4) 11.

Angelica

Basil
Bergamot
Black pepper
Blue Cypress

Cardamom
Cedarwood
Celery Seed
Cinnamon Bark
Cistus
Clary Sage
Clove
Copaiba
Cypress

Dill
Dorado Azul

Elemi
Eucalyptus blue
Eucalyptus Radiata

Fennel
Frankincense

Galbanum
Geranium
German Chamomile
Ginger
Goldenrod
Grapefruit

Helichrystum
Hinoki
Hong Kuai

Hyssop
Idaho Balsam Fir
Idaho Blue Spruce

Jade Lemon
Jasmine
Juniper

Laurus Nobilis
Lavender
Ledum
Lemon
Lemon Myrtle
Lemongrass
Lime

Manuka
Marjoram
Mastrante
Melaleuca (Tea Tree Oil)
Melissa (Lemon balm)
Mountain Savory
Myrrh
Myrtle

Neroli
Northern Lights Black
Spruce
Nutmeg

Ocotea
Orange
Oregano

Palmarosa
Palo Santo
Patchouli

Peppermint
Petitgrain
Pine

Ravintsara
Rose
Rosemary
Royal Hawaiian
Sandalwood

Sacred Frankincense
Sage (Salva)
Spearmint
Spikenard

Tangerine
Tarragon
Tea Tree (Melaleuca)
Thyme
Tsoga

Valerian
Vetiver

Wintergreen

Xiang Mao

Ylang Ylang

Table 1.1 Varieties of essential oils

CHAPTER 2

ESSENTIAL OIL PLANTS

E xtracting essential oils from their parent botanicals is addressed in Chapter 3 but central to this issue is the importance of the quality of the parent plants. In Chapter 1, it was stated that the important factors determining the quality of all plants and trees used as sources of essential oils include where they are grown and all the environmental conditions existing during the growth period. This horticultural principle is well-established with gardeners and agronomists. It was also noted in Chapter 1 that the taste and characteristics of olive oil and wines likewise are markedly affected by where the olives and wine grapes were grown as well as the local climactic and environmental conditions.

It follows, therefore, that the properties and characteristics of nominally the same essential oil from a named plant source will be modified, and often markedly influenced in characteristics such as aroma and health benefits, by the growth factors outlined previously. This is an important principle in the production of essential oils. When extracted oils from different source materials are compounded or mixed together, the resultant essential oil can often be unsatisfactory. It is the careful adherence to the cultivation of plant materials that distinguishes Young Living essential oils from those of many competitors and, particularly, from cheaper products that are claimed to be 100% pure. Unfortunately, many so-called "pure" essential oils may contain diluents and adulterants. Young Living has well-controlled and carefully husbanded orchards and plant farms all over the world to ensure the highest quality for their products.

In today's health conscious world, consumers are encouraged to buy *organic* fruit and vegetables as well as poultry, eggs and meats that are organically grown/raised. The higher price of "organic" foodstuffs is justified by vague comments like "they are healthier", "better for you", "are better tasting" but such statements are rarely supported or even explained but few people understand what the term "organic" means.

In Chapter 1, reference was made to "organic", a term that has two meanings or applications in science. The first is in *Organic Chemistry*, a major subdiscipline in chemistry and encompasses the scientific study of the structure, properties and reactions of the various forms of matter (i.e., chemicals) that contain carbon atoms. In other words, this is the field of chemistry dealing with what are known organic compounds and which include everything from lubricating oils, plastics, petrochemicals, pharmaceuticals, solvents and resins as well as essential oils.

In the agribusiness, notably the food industry, the term *organic* refers to foods farmed using practices that promote balance and biodiversity throughout the environment. Thus, "organic" foods and botanicals are grown without the use of pesticides, herbicides and artificial fertilizers. Further, organic foods should not have been treated with or contain synthetic food additives and have not been exposed to solvents or irradiation other than natural sunlight. Organic farming of animals and poultry adheres to the same restrictions when they were raised and warrants that they were not treated with antibiotics or other growth stimulants and that they were not exposed to radiation or pesticides in their food. The limitations imposed by claims of organic farming are important because, unfortunately, agrochemicals, notably pesticides, are dangerous and can be toxic, as mentioned in Chapter 1. Consequently, the common practice of parents insisting that children (and adults) should wash fruit and vegetables before eating them makes sense if needless and unwanted exposure to toxic chemicals on the skins of fruits and vegetables is to be avoided. It is for this reason that responsible producers of essential oils like Young Living insist on organic-based farming principles for the plants grown to make their products.

At first glance, extracting essential oils from organically-grown botanicals does not appear to be an important or even necessary refinement. However, the fact that the "organic" source plants were grown without artificial, notably chemical, agents means that the flowers, leaves and other components from which essential oils are extracted are free from synthetic materials both on their surfaces and within their structures. This is a very important consideration because most pesticides, herbicides and, indeed, some chemical fertilizers can be toxic, as noted above, and many of these compounds are allergenic, i.e., they can be allergens. Allergens cause allergic skin reactions such as itching, hives and other rashes as well as classic allergic reactions like sneezing, runny noses, watery eyes and wheezing or other respiratory problems. In fact, according to the American Academy of Dermatology, fragrances are the leading cause of cosmetic contact dermatitis. As a health problem, this sensitivity alone affects more than 2 million people in the United States, and it appears that sensitivity is on the rise.

Table 2.1 indicates the essential oils that most frequently cause allergic reactions or other sensitivity issues although such effects are not common. The prevalence of adverse reactions to essential oils extracted from non-organically grown botanical sources or to essential oils that are blended with diluents or those containing adulterants and solvent residues may be much greater. It is likely, however, that organically grown, 100% pure, essential oils may contain far fewer allergens because they are wholly natural and free of such allergens.

Table 2.1 Essential Oils that May Elicit Sensitivity Reactions

Basil	Lemongrass	Spruce
Camphor*	Oregano	Thyme
Cassia	Pine	Vetiver
Cinnamon	Rosemary	White fir
Fir Needle	Sage	Wintergreen

*This oil is not available from Young Living

Clearly, using botanicals grown under organic conditions as sources of essential oils is important because these plant-derived aromatic compounds are present in a great number of perfumes, body cremes and fragrances. Purity, absence of herbicides and insecticides as well as solvent residues or dilution of the essential oil with extraneous material such as cheaper vegetable oils and coconut oil are all things that must be considered when anything is applied to the skin or even inhaled as in aromatherapy.

There is another benefit to organically-grown plants such as fruit and vegetables. Very recent research[5] performed at the Teagasc Ashtown Food Research Centre in Carlow, Ireland has shown that the content of two types of flavonoids are significantly higher (by 10-50%) in "organic" onions than conventionally grown ones. This finding is very significant in that flavonoids may protect consumers against many chronic health conditions such cardiovascular disease, diabetes and cancer.

It should be noted that the National Organic Standards Board requires that food (and flower) producers use organically grown seeds, annual seedlings, and planting stock. Non-organically produced, untreated seeds and planting stock may be used to produce an organic crop when an equivalent organically-produced variety is not commercially available. Because Young Living grows much of its own botanicals, their plants are all grown from organically-grown seeds. Before discussing botanicals grown for essential oils, it might be useful to briefly review seeds and seedlings. Figure 2.1 is a schematic representation of the overall process involved in growing plants as sources of essential oils.

---

5   Alla Katnelson; Organic onions are richer in flavonoids. Chemical and Engineering News (2017) 95 (27) Page 8 quoting data from J. Agric. Food Chem. (2017) 10: 1021.

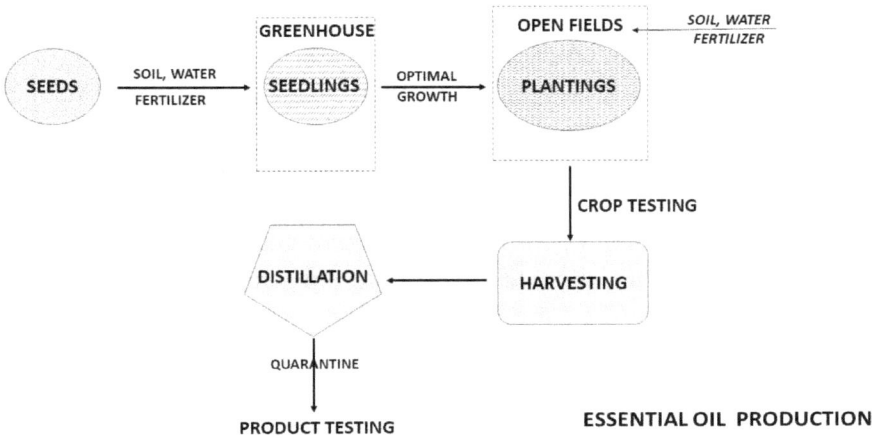

Figure 2.1 Schematic diagram of crop farming for essential oils.

Seed Germination and Seedling Growth

Commercial growers of organic botanicals and seed producers try to mimic nature by growing their products with a minimum of external inputs such as pesticides, herbicides and the like, ideally starting with organic seeds and seedlings. Thus, growers spend a great deal of time and energy learning as much as possible about the biology of the plants they intend to grow and to ecological systems pertaining to their crops, and then apply this knowledge to their farming practice.

Viable seeds are living entities. For germination (the initial growth of a seed) to occur, they must contain healthy embryonic tissue and, therefore, they contain both an embryo as well as food reserves within the seed coat. Seeds will start to germinate when both the soil moisture content and the temperature conditions are right for the process to initiate. Each seed type has individual needs and characteristic temperature ranges for germination. Depending upon the plant, provided the temperature is above a minimum range (30-60°F/0-16°C) and below a maximum range (85-100°F/29-38°C) with an optimal range of (40-95°F/4-35°C), germination generally is rapid and uniform. Under low or high temperature conditions, i.e. outside of the optimum range, seeds may go into dormancy and not germinate.

Although temperature is important, soil moisture content and soil aeration are vital. In particular, there must be good seed-to-soil contact and a fine-textured seedbed for there to be good gas exchange between the germinating embryo and the soil for optimal germination. Soil aeration of the growing medium allows respiration of the seeds because, like all living organisms, they need to take in oxygen from the air and exhale carbon dioxide (CO_2). Not only that, the exhaled CO_2 must also dissipate (i.e., migrate or diffuse) away from the growing seed to protect the seeds from suffocating. Seed suffocation typically can occur when they are planted in compacted, water-saturated, or very dense soil because any of these soil conditions can obstruct or limit dissipation of the exhaled CO_2.

Whereas seedlings require light to strengthen and grow properly, the situation is different for seeds. Most seeds germinate best in the dark although there are some that do require light for germination to occur.

It is worth noting that viable seeds do not always germinate because they can enter a dormancy period which prevents germination even under optimal environmental and growth conditions. It is possible, however, that even dormant seeds will germinate over time and this staggered germination appears to be nature's way of ensuring that at least some seeds will survive if there are sudden and possibly adverse changes in the weather or the growing conditions. This is particularly true for seeds that germinate in the spring, i.e. when the cold weather should have broken, although as most people know, sudden cold snaps often occur during the spring, wreaking havoc on seeds and seedlings. Professional growers and nurseries have established techniques for bringing seeds out of dormancy but their approaches to the different types of dormancy are beyond the scope of this book. Nevertheless, professional growers want seeds to germinate as quickly as possible because uneven germination can cause problems, particularly if greenhouse space is limited and is needed for germination and seedling growth of other plant types. Accordingly, growers will aim to customize the conditions using special growth media and careful temperature, air flow and moisture control to optimize uniform germination.

Seed germination is a three-stage process. The first stage is imbibition or uptake of water by the seed which causes its coating to soften and swell. Imbibition is then followed by a lag phase during which the internal physiology of the seed is activated to encourage cellular respiration, initiate formation of proteins and start metabolization of stored foods. In the third and final stage, cells within the seed start to elongate and divide, and then the radicle (the primary root) starts to emerge from the seed and anchor the plant to the ground. As the root absorbs water, the shoot emerges from the seed and the seedlings start to develop.

After the shoot emerges, the seedling grows slowly, the storage tissues of the seed shrink as their contents are consumed and the plant develops a branched root system, known as the taproot. Then leaves develop and photosynthesize light into energy so that the plant seedling grows and develops. Again, moisture and temperature must be controlled to ensure optimal growth, and this is best achieved by having both seed germination and seedling development take place in a greenhouse.

A final step must be taken before seedlings are planted in the field and that is to progressively expose them to the conditions they will experience outside. This process, known as *hardening off*, stimulates the plants to accumulate carbohydrate and nutrient reserves and strengthens cell walls by exposing the plants to daytime/nighttime temperature and light fluctuations, increased air movement and wind, reduced watering as well as full light during daylight hours.

Another important factor in seed germination and seedling growth is the soil quality, notably its mineral content and it is known that the mineral content of plants, notably fruits and vegetables, depends on how and where they were grown. Thus, soil mineral content is important to plant quality, but this is a characteristic that was difficult to assess until a Florida agricultural engineer, Dr. Carey A. Reams, developed what is known as the Brix chart back in the 1970s. This chart, which covers most common fruits, vegetables and forage crops, is used with a device known as a refractometer (see Appendix A) to guide growers on the quality of their plantings. If the Brix reading for a plant is poor, then the grower can adopt measures to improve the quality of his crop such as providing fertilizer. Clearly, growers that aim to optimize the quality of plants for essential oils will undertake Brix measurements on a routine basis throughout seedling growth.

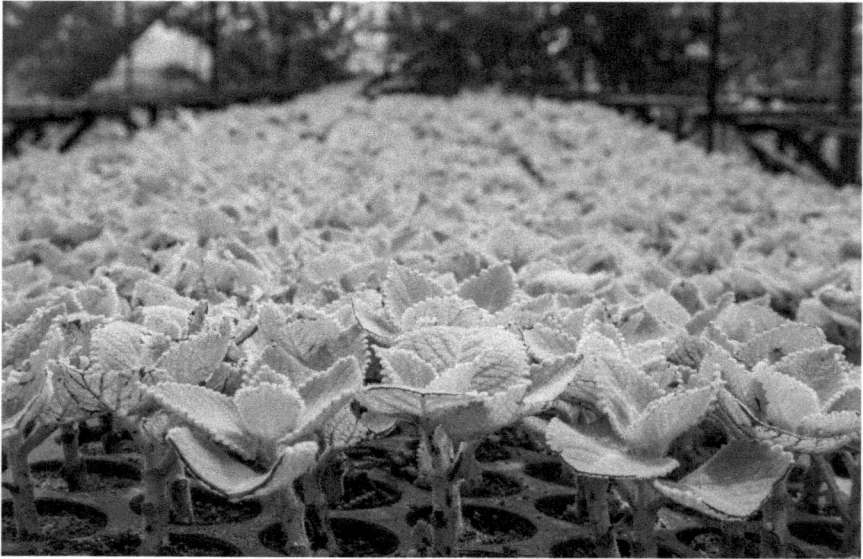

**Figure 2.2 Seedlings growing in a greenhouse
(Courtesy of Young Living)**

After hardening off, the seedlings are carefully transplanted into the field and spaced appropriately such that there is adequate room for each seedling to growth into a healthy plant. Thereafter, irrigation, weed control and fertilization with natural fertilizers are instituted until the plants are harvested.

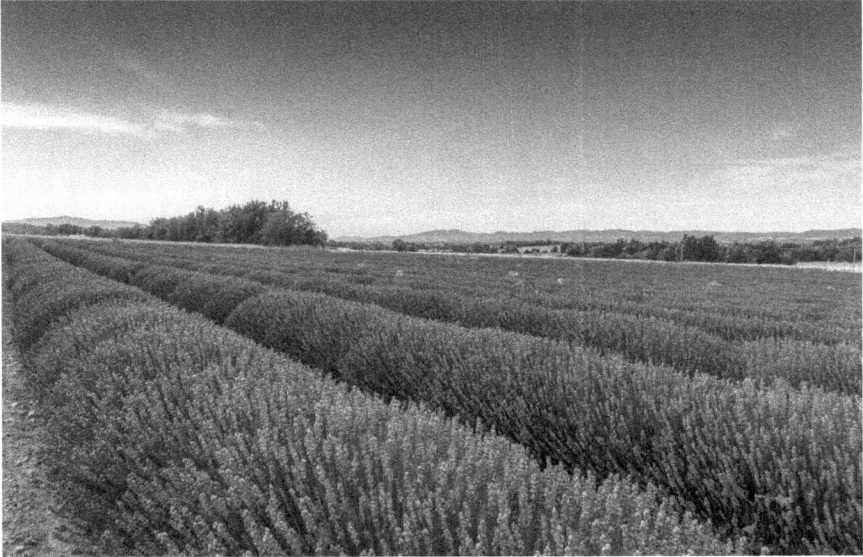

**Figure 2.3 Field of maturing plants before
harvesting (Courtesy of Young Living)**

It should be obvious from the above, that a great deal of time, skill and effort as well as considerable resources must be invested to grow the botanicals used as sources of essential oils. It is also understandable why Young Living takes great pride in proclaiming that it truly is a "From the Ground Up" Company and that all its products are 100% pure and grown under conservational and ecologically benign conditions.

It should also be noted that plant quality, and its essential oil, is also dependent upon the harvesting method that is used and, indeed, when in the growth cycle the plants are harvested. If harvesting is performed too early, or too late, plant and essential oil quality are adversely affected. Consequently, growers will measure the Brix value (see Appendix A) of their plants almost on a daily basis towards the end of the growing season to ensure that harvesting is performed at the precise time that plant quality is at its highest.

Two final factors within the germination, growth and harvesting cycle are the harvesting method and post-harvest handling of the plants. Hand-picking is obviously "kinder" to the plants and reduces inclusion of dirt, insects and other extraneous matter in the collected crop, but is highly labor intensive. Mechanical harvesting is faster, and far more efficient but other matter can also be entrained in the crop. The actual method adopted for a particular plant crop will be determined by the plant, where it is grown and the field size where it is to be harvested. Following harvesting, the gathered crop may or may not be dried.

Plant drying can have significant benefits such as minimizing soil contamination, mold growth and fermentation. It can also extend the period between harvesting and distillation because the risk of plant degradation is kept to a minimum. Drying correspondingly reduces distillation time by permitting more plant material to be placed in the still at one time. Various drying methods are used, typically open-air drying, laying out in vented drying barns or even oven drying. On the other hand, there are certain disadvantages to plant drying. Care must be exercised during any drying operation, particularly when using heat or through sunlight, to avoid damage to the plant material and consequent loss of essential oil through evaporation or degradation. Accordingly, drying is not generally performed on harvested material, especially with more sensitive plants, to ensure optimal yield and quality of the essential oil.

Essential Oils: Synthetics *vs*. Natural

In the context of pure and organic essential oils, it might be useful to look at why "natural" essential oils are far preferable to synthetic oils. There is no question that nominally the same synthetic products cost less, often markedly so, than the natural products. The classic example of this price differential is when one compares the prices of organic fruit and vegetables in a supermarket to those of the same products grown under ordinary farming conditions, that is, when the crops have been sprayed with artificial fertilizers, herbicides and pesticides to encourage growth and higher yields. However, the differences in taste and texture between "ordinary" and "organically grown" fruit and vegetables are usually obvious.

Essential oils are extracted from plants and there is a cost, in fact a high cost, associated with the extraction process, packaging and everything else involved in the production of essential oils and the multitude of products containing them. Let's look at nootkatone, a citrus molecule that is the main chemical component responsible for the smell and flavor of the grapefruit. It is an effective repellent/insecticide that is environmentally friendly because it is a volatile essential oil that does not persist in the environment. Nootkatone is nontoxic to humans and is an approved food additive commonly used in foods, cosmetics, and pharmaceuticals. Extracting nootkatone from grapefruit requires about 400,000 lb. (200 tons) of grapefruit to produce 1 lb. (454 grams) or about $80,000/lb. if grapefruit can be purchased at only 20¢/lb. In marked contrast, synthetic nootkatone only costs about $2000 per pound, i.e. a fraction of the cost of the natural product as well as requiring considerably less material for its manufacture. Although some experts claim that there is no difference between synthetic and natural essential oils, it must be stressed that no natural essential oil has only a single component. In fact, plant-derived essential oils contain several and often dozens of different components that comprise the *essence* of the parent botanical.

Clearly differences between synthetic and naturally-derived oils can be quite marked. A simple example of this is that there are readily distinguishable differences in the taste, consistency and "feel" between premium olive oils from, say, France, Spain, Greece and Turkey but why are there such differences? After all, olive oil comes from the same botanical material, namely olives. The differences come from within the olives themselves because the composition of each berry, the "chemical" make-up of the olive, reflects the conditions under which it was grown, notably climate, soil and irrigation to name but a few factors. Each of these factors imparts a fractional but definite effect on the final berry (and the resultant olive oil) but they all work together synergistically. In other words, every small and even fractional influence working in concert with each other is greater than simply adding together the various individual effects. These synergistic effects are well-known to chefs the world over when they add small amounts of different spices and herbs to create a gourmet meal.

The same effect occurs with wholly natural essential oils. Although both natural and synthetic oils may have the same major component or components, it is the fractional ingredients that make all the difference in the quality and effectiveness of the natural essential oil. It is hard to believe that an essential oil manufactured in a chemical plant or laboratory will contain the same or even comparable minor components to an essential oil extracted from organically-grown botanicals. Further, it is difficult to accept that that the laboratory-created product has properties that even approach, let alone equal, the wholly natural essential oil.

Botanical Sources of Essential Oils

The incredible array of pure essential oils marketed by Young Living, see Table 1.1, indicates that these products have been extracted from a wide diversity of flowers, herbs, bushes and trees. In addition to the pure oils listed in Table 1.1, Young Living also produces many different oil blends formulated for aromatherapeutic, massage, diffusion and nutritional applications. These specialized products and formulations, and their uses, are discussed elsewhere in this book. The important thing is that all these products are 100% pure and natural, and do not contain any adulterants or synthetic products.

Most of Young Living's essential oils are extracted from the flowers, leaves and tree parts that are familiar in many parts of the United States. Closer inspection of Table 1.1, however, reveals that many of the essential oil plants are not native to the United States and, accordingly, are imported from overseas. As such, importation of foreign plants into the U.S.A. is subject to the Lacey Act[6,7] and Young Living is meticulous in complying with this regulation on importing plants. Further, the fact that those foreign-sourced plants and trees are grown under strict conservation and ecologically-controlled conditions in dedicated plantations and farms ensures the highest purity products. In this context, compliance with the Lacey Act requires identification

---

6   The Lacey Act of 1900 is a U.S. conservation law that prohibits trade in wildlife, fish and plants that have been illegally taken, possessed, transported, or sold. The Lacey Act was amended on May 22, 2008, when the Food, Conservation and Energy Act of 2008 widened its protection to a broader range of plants and plant products Accordingly, it is now unlawful to import, export, transport, sell, receive, acquire, or purchase any plant in violation of the laws of the United States or any foreign law that protects plants.

7   von Fraunhofer J A, Joshi RK. Essential oils and the legislative landscape. American Journal of Essential Oils and Natural Products (2019) 7(1): 01-06.

of the grower, farming conditions, harvesting protocols and shipping practices to ensure all U.S. and foreign laws are satisfied.

The other regulatory law governing products in this area is CITES[8], which is one of the largest and oldest International conservation and sustainable use agreements in existence. CITES provides varying degrees of protection to more than 35,000 species of fauna and flora against over-exploitation through international trade but National participation is voluntary. and countries that are bound by the Convention are known as Parties. Although CITES is legally binding on the Parties, it does not replace national laws so that in the U.S.A. for example, the U.S. Lacey Act is the primary regulatory instrument for any plants or wildlife imported into, or exported from, the U.S.A. Consequently, claims by some essential oil companies that they are CITES-compliant carries far less weight with regard to conservation efforts than compliance with the Lacey Act as practiced by Young Living.

Another thing that stands out from Table 1.1 is that a wide range of botanicals are used as sources of essential oils and the diversity of plants, notably flowers, trees and shrubs, means that different extraction procedures often are used to obtain the oils. Further, different parts of each plant are involved in the extraction process. Clearly, extracting lavender or geranium oil is going to be far different from extracting essential oil from, say, Idaho blue spruce or cinnamon bark. If nothing else, it is obviously easier to handle a wheelbarrow full of flowers than one filled with tree branches. Not only that, although the overall extraction process, namely distillation (see Chapter 3), is broadly the same regardless of plant source, the extraction conditions involved with trees and shrubs are going to be markedly different from those used with flowers. This is where the art, science and skill of the essential oil extraction artisan comes into play.

---

8   CITES (the Convention on International Trade in Endangered Species of Wild Fauna and Flora, also known as the Washington Convention) is a multilateral treaty to protect endangered animals and plants.

CHAPTER 3

EXTRACTING
ESSENTIAL OILS

E ssential oils have been used in cosmetics, perfumes and for
medicinal purposes for thousands of years, in fact almost since
the dawn of civilization. Just when and how essential oils were
first extracted from plants is unknown but the extraction methods in
current use have a venerable history.

Although there are records of which plants were used as botanical sources, there are few details available on the actual methods
used for extracting essentials oils. What we do know about essential
oil extraction can be gleaned from Mycenean (Ancient Greek/Bronze
Age) tablets and Assyrian records in the 13th Century BC. More information was detailed in the 4th Century BC writings of Theophratus[9].
Several centuries later in the 1st Century AD, Dioscorides[10] wrote *De
Materia Medica*, a pharmacopoeia of herbs and the medicines that can
be obtained from them. During the same time period also in the 1st

---

9   Theophratus was a Greek native of Eresos in Lesbos and a successor to Aristotle
    in the Peripatetic school and who also studied in Plato's school.

10 Pedanius Dioscorides was a Greek physician, pharmacologist and botanist who
    wrote a 5-volume encyclopedia of herbal medicine and related medicinal sub-
    stances known as *De Materia Medica*. This collection of knowledge was widely
    read for more than 1,500 years.

Century AD but in a different region, Pliny the Elder, the Roman author, naturalist and natural philosopher, wrote *Naturalis Historia*, a compendium describing aromatic plants and areas where they grew.

Apparently, a variety of methods were used in ancient times for extracting essential oils from their botanical sources and many of these approaches are still used today. However, most oils are now extracted on a commercial scale by distillation. The basic distillation process is often combined with the injection of steam into the distillation vessel or "still" to help release the oil from the plant, as discussed below. Other extraction processes include squeezing (expression), solvent or oil extraction, leaching out the oil with animal fat and tapping of the tree trunk, the latter method being used for frankincense and myrrh, the oils of antiquity.

It appears that the ancients used a basic extraction process that involved chopping up the flowers, leaves, branches, fruits and aromatic resins exuded from certain trees and then pressing them. Thereafter, the plant material was steeped in hot and cold oil to release and absorb the aromatic compounds. Apparently, the ancient Greeks used linseed oil, the Israelites used olive oil whereas sesame oil was used in Mesopotamia while the ancient Egyptians used animal fats. Regardless of the actual extraction medium used, the aroma-infused oil was decanted into alabaster or lead containers and allowed to cool and settle for a few days. Then the oil was boiled, strained and transferred into smaller containers ready for use or trading. This extraction process is the basis for what is known by the French term *enfleurage*.

Enfleurage

Enfleurage could be the oldest known method of extracting and preserving the fragrances of flowering plants (botanicals) and has been used since pre-biblical times. Enfleurage is also often referred to as "maceration", the term for the softening of a solid plant by soaking so that its internal fibers separate, and the delicate or highly volatile floral essence can be leached out.

One traditional approach to fragrance extraction, known as *hot* enfleurage and which is clearly based on the ancient extraction methods, involves melting solid fats in a pot and then stirring the botanicals into it. When all fragrance has been leached out from the flowers, the spent plants are strained off and replaced with fresh material until the fat is saturated with fragrance.

The *cold* enfleurage process was developed in Southern France during the 18th century for producing high-grade concentrates. In this process, a large-framed plate of glass, known as a "chassis", is smeared with a layer of rendered and clarified animal fat, usually tallow or lard[11], and allowed to set. Then the botanical matter, usually petals but might also be whole flowers, is placed on the fat so that its scent can diffuse into the fat over 1-3 days but sometimes over a period of weeks. This process is then repeated by replacing spent botanicals with fresh ones until the fat has reached the required degree of fragrance saturation.

In both the hot and cold enfleurage processes, the final product is fat saturated with fragrance and which is known as "enfleurage pomade" or scented ointment. The pomade may either be sold as is or it can be soaked in alcohol (ethanol) to leach out the aroma compounds. After separating out any residual fat, the alcohol is allowed to evaporate off, leaving behind the "absolute" botanical, that is, *the essential oil.* Traditionally, the spent fat, which still retains a fair amount of fragrance, was used to produce soap. It is possible that the perfumes and precious oils mentioned in several places within the bible were obtained by the enfleurage process and, given that this is such a labor-intensive process, that alone would make them precious.

Despite the inefficiency and cost in terms of manpower, enfleurage until comparatively recently was the only method of extracting fragrances from delicate flowers which might otherwise be denatured (destroyed) in the high temperatures used in distillation. Now, more efficient extraction techniques such as solvent extraction and supercritical fluid extraction using a liquified gas such as carbon dioxide (CO_2) are used for delicate botanicals such as jasmine and tuberose.

---

11   Two rendered and clarified animal fats, lard and tallow, are used in enfleurage. Lard is fat from the abdomen of a pig whereas tallow comes from beef or mutton. They are rendered by slow heating with a small amount of water and then straining off the clarified fat which solidifies at room temperature.

Nevertheless, enfleurage apparently is still used in rural areas in various parts of the world.

It would appear, however, that essential oils were also extracted in ancient times by crude distillation methods although, again, few details are available on the processes involved. Also, it is not clear whether enfleurage or distillation was favored back in ancient times or, indeed, which extraction method came first.

Distillation

The basic concept of distillation is that the liquid contained within the still (the distillation vessel or heating chamber) is boiled to form vapor. The released vapor rises to the top of the still where it passes from the head or cap down into the condenser where it cools back to a liquid and is collected in the receiver. Although often thought of as a modern process, distillation is actually a very old method of extracting essential oils from botanicals and a few words on the history of the subject might be useful here.

Historical records indicate that the art of distillation was described by Herodotus at about 400 BC and then described again, some 50 years later, by Aristotle. However, the discovery of earthenware distillation apparatus dating back to about 3000 BC suggests that steam distillation to extract essential oils may have been practiced for around 5000 years and possibly even longer. What is not known with any degree of certainty is which oils were extracted and for what purpose, although both medicines and perfumery (and possibly liquors) are likely candidates as products of this ancient practice.

Archeological findings and written records indicate that a degree of science crept into the then rather crude distillation techniques with the activities of Greek chemists in Alexandria in the 1st Century AD and, at around the same time, in China during the Han Dynasty (100-200 AD). However, it is quite possible that the primary purpose of such distillation techniques was to produce alcoholic beverages, purified water, so-called "divine water" and medicinal fluids rather than just to extract essential oils from plants.

Since those very early days, sparse written records indicate that distillation of water, essential oils and probably liquors has continued until the present day. Early written references to distillation include the works of Arabian chemists in the 1st and 2nd Centuries AD and, notably, Zosimos of Panopolis. The latter, who lived in the Southern part of Roman Egypt at the end of the 3rd and beginning of the 4th century AD, wrote the oldest known books on alchemy. His enthusiasm for alchemy suggests that distillation was a "black art" although Zosimos had a clear understanding of the requirements for effective distillation.

His distillation equipment comprised a still pot (known as the cucurbit), a vapor collecting cap or head to the still (known as the anbik), a condensing tube and a receiver. In the Zosimos system, the liquid contained within the still pot or cucurbit is boiled by an external heat source to form vapor. The vapor is collected by the anbik and directed into the air-cooled condenser. As the cooled vapor descends the condenser, it reverts to the liquid state and is collected in the receiver.

These separate elements or components of ancient stills are basically the same as those used in chemical laboratories by chemistry students the world over and in modern distillation equipment. With early stills, condensers appear to have been air-cooled whereas laboratory-scale set-ups and modern systems commonly use water-cooling of the condenser to aid condensation of the vapor released from the still.

Sporadic comments about rudimentary distillation are to be found in writings from the Dark Ages (the early Middle Ages). However, more refined distillation techniques appear to have been developed in China during the Jin (12th – 13th centuries), Southern Song (10th – 13th centuries) and Yuan (13th - 14th centuries) dynasties. Since then, of course, distillation methods have become far more efficient, better controlled and based upon science rather than the earlier trial-and-error methodologies. In addition to the greater efficiency and through-put performance of modern distilleries, superior construction materials and manufacturing technology have greatly reduced the inclusion of impurities in essential oils due accretions from the processing equipment.

Large-scale Distillation

Nowadays, the commonest commercial method of obtaining essential oils is by distillation with the source material being heated in a closed container or still to drive off or liberate the desired compound (the essential oil) from the botanical source (usually seeds or flowers but also leaves, branches and bark). The released gaseous material is then passed from the still head into an externally cooled tube where the vapor cools and condenses into a liquid to be collected in a suitable container. This approach is often referred to as classic or simple distillation. A more detailed discussion of the distillation process is to be found elsewhere.[12] Classically, distillation is how alcoholic beverages (liquors) such as whisky, gin, brandy, rum and vodka are produced.

Young Living favors distillation for extracting essential oils because it allows greater control of the overall extraction process. Although the basic processes involved in distillation are much the same regardless of the material being processed, the extraction conditions required for trees and shrubs are markedly different to those used with flowers. As with any physical or chemical process involving fragile, valuable and heat-sensitive materials, the artisan performing essential oil extraction must exercise sound scientific/technological knowledge and a great deal of skill. Because the extraction procedure involves heat, there must be careful control of the distillation process to ensure that the source plants and the extracted essential oil are not subject to thermal damage. Further, the distillation equipment must be non-reactive, e.g. the still and every component must be constructed using stainless steel or other non-corrodible material to avoid contamination of the product.

Steam distillation, often referred to as *hydrodistillation*, is used to separate heat-sensitive components from their botanical source. It involves passing steam into the plant matter in the still, causing heating of the mixture and some of it to vaporize. This vapor is cooled and condensed into two liquid fractions, one principally water and the other the extracted matter. Sometimes the fractions are collected separately or, because they have different densities, they separate themselves into discrete layers in the receiver. This separation effect occurs when flowers (botanicals) are steam distilled and the distillation products are the essential oil and a water-based (aqueous) distillate. In common with vacuum distillation (see below), steam distillation is a method of achieving distillation at temperatures lower than the normal boiling point of the component to be separated. It often is used when the

12   J. A. von Fraunhofer. *Essential Oils. A concise guide.* Kindle Direct Publishing/ Amazon (2017).

component to be distilled is immiscible (incapable of mixing) with, and chemically unreactive, with water.

Vacuum or reduced pressure distillation is used to separate components in a mixture when the components have high boiling points. Lowering the pressure within the still lowers boiling points of the liquids inside the heating chamber. In most other respects, vacuum distillation is essentially the same as simple and steam distillation, but it is particularly useful when the normal boiling point of a compound is higher than its decomposition temperature, i.e., the compound to be separated is subject to thermal degradation. Since vacuum distillation operates at lower temperatures than those used in conventional or steam distillation, there is a reduced risk of product degradation, an important factor in extracting heat-sensitive essential oils. Although equipment and operating costs are higher than for simple or steam distillation, the overall process improves separation efficiency and actually lowers the cost of the essential oil because of greater still capacity, higher yields and superior product purity.

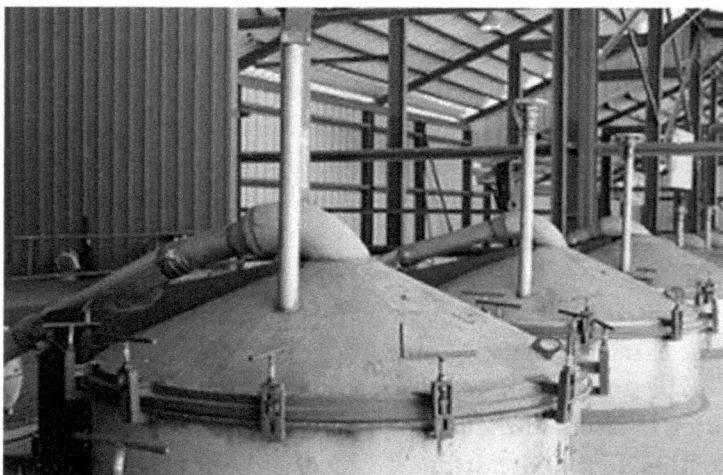

Figure 3.1 Large scale industrial distillation (Courtesy of Young Living)

Obviously, given the scale of the operation at Young Living, very large stills are operated under strict process controls and all distillation units were manufactured using inert materials. Because the source botanicals are seasonal, the distillation systems are run intermittently but these breaks in operation enable the operators to regularly clean and maintain the systems to ensure the clarity and absence of sediments in the extracted essential oil.

CHAPTER 4

ESSENTIAL OILS IN THE ANCIENT WORLD

E ssential oils and perfumes have been important to man for millennia, making almost incalculable contributions to civilization as we know it. They have been used in worship, cosmetics, as food flavorants and in medicine since time immemorial.

Ancient botanical sources of essential oils

Historically, most essential oils and then their derived perfumes were obtained from herbs, flowers, bushes or trees although a few were developed from animal sources. Many of these aromatics were harvested by wounding or "tapping" trees and the base or principal ingredient for the perfume either trickled out or simply oozed from the bark wound. This method, albeit somewhat refined, is still used for harvesting the sap from maple trees to make maple syrup and to get the venerable essential oils myrrh and frankincense from their source trees. Another way to get oleoresins was by "tapping" the accumulation or accretion of substances beneath a bruise in the tree bark. These oleoresinous[13]

---

13 *Oleoresins* are naturally occurring semi-solid mixtures of a resin dissolved in an essential oil and/or a fatty oil obtained from certain plants. They are also known as balsams.

substances were not the sap of the tree and despite their chemical complexity, they fell into three main groups:

1.   Resins: insoluble in water but often soluble in alcohol,
2.   Gums: insoluble in alcohol but capable of absorbing water to form a mucilage[14], and
3.   Oleoresins and balsams: solutions of resins in volatile oils and a primary source of perfumes.

The total quantity of the different resins, gums and balsams used in antiquity was enormous, both in the variety of resins and the amount of material used. The most important of these oleoresins were frankincense, myrrh and turpentine, all of which were obtained from the trees of those names. Of these, myrrh was the most widely used although the proportion used for medical purposes is unknown. Interestingly, the bark of the myrrh tree apparently cracks spontaneously, allowing the oleoresin to trickle out and eventually harden into a reddish-brown mass. Myrrh has a characteristic bitter taste and its name derives from the Hebrew and Arabic word *murr* for bitter. In contrast, frankincense was traditionally collected by making longitudinal incisions through the bark and allowing the white gum to come to the surface where it solidified. Within 1-2 weeks, the white lump dried into an amber-colored oleoresin gum that ignites easily and burns to give off a pleasant smell (i.e., incense). The importance of frankincense is underscored by the fact that Queen Hatshepsut of Egypt sent a fleet to the ancient kingdom of Punt, an Egyptian trading partner, to bring back whole frankincense trees in the 15th Century BC. It appears that the transplanted trees did not survive, and similar expeditions were undertaken for another 300 years, apparently with little success.

Historical records of the extraction of essential oils from plants in early times are somewhat imprecise but, based on Mycenean tablets, it is possible that the method known as *enfleurage* or maceration (see Chapter 3) was relatively common. Although enfleurage was practiced back in ancient times, and is still used today in Europe and elsewhere, records indicate that distillation also was practiced thousands of years

---

14   Mucilage is a viscous or gelatinous solution from plant roots, seeds, etc. The term mucilage is used for medicines and, commonly, when referring to adhesives.

ago, as discussed in Chapter 3. Interestingly, despite its antiquity, distillation is now the most common commercial method of obtaining essential oils and has been widely used since the early centuries of this millennium. Distillation is a far more efficient and less labor-intensive for extracting essential oils from botanical sources than maceration/enfleurage.

Although the approaches to extracting essential oils from their parent plants in the distant past were roughly comparable to today's methods, the processing back then was considerably less efficient than is possible today, especially with respect to distillation. Lower yields and questionable product purity were likely the norm for oils in antiquity compared to the present day due, at least in part, to impurities and contaminants in the distillate. These impurities are the result of several factors, including inefficient distillation methods, the accretion of sediments, residues and other matter in the still and in other parts of the distillation equipment. Poor temperature control during heating of the botanical matter during the extraction process would also have lowered extraction efficiency and added to the impurity burden of the extracted oils. In other words, essential oils available to the ancients were likely far less pure than the products now available from companies like Young Living with their precise control of the extraction process and the use of corrosion-resistant materials for the construction of their stills and associated equipment. However, it should be stated that, like the botanicals used by Young Living, the plants used by the ancients as sources of essential oils were undoubtedly grown under organic conditions so that they were free of herbicides and pesticides.

Essential Oils and Perfumes

Essential oils and perfumes have been inextricably entwined for millennia. The word *perfume* had a far broader meaning in Ancient Times than today and encompassed not just perfume but also incense, spices, ointments (unguents[15]) and medicines. The origin of the word perfume is thought to be the Latin phrase *per furnum*, which means "by or through fire or an oven" and is probably a reference to distillation. On the other hand, it could also be a reference to the spiritual role of

---

15   The word unguent derives from the Latin word *unguentum* for an ointment.

perfumes in the sacrificial fires which were intended to provide food for the "gods" who would starve without these offerings. At about the same time (i.e., 3-4000 years ago), and probably even earlier than that, "perfumes" and aromatic oils were deemed to be basic necessities in life. There are comments by historians that slave laborers (and probably the Israelites) in Ancient Egypt sometimes went on strike because their food was bad, and they had no *ointment* to improve the taste.

There are numerous references to perfumes and oils in the Bible, the Talmud and other classical writings. Records clearly show that spices, aromatic oils and perfumes were known throughout the ancient world and were coveted by kings, princes and wealthy citizens in many cultures from the earliest periods of recorded history.

Production of perfume and essential oils was previously mentioned in Chapter 3. Ancient sources from as early as the 13th Century BC, notably Mycenean tablets, Assyrian records, Egyptian papyri, engravings on tomb walls and scriptures all contain recipes for the preparation of perfumes and these writings often detailed the ingredients and tools required to make perfumes. The ingredients used to make perfume included essential oils such as spikenard[16], saffron, henna, sweet cane and cinnamon as well as myrrh and frankincense.

Because extracting essential oils and making perfumes and unguents involved considerable effort as well as great skill, perfumers had high social standing and were held in great regard. Further, because perfumes, essential oils and fragrant spices were precious commodities and much in demand in antiquity, they sometimes were regarded as more valuable than gold and silver. This would explain why the bible indicates that the Judaean kings kept oils, perfumes and spices in treasure houses and the Queen of Sheba brought camels laden with spices (and, presumably, perfumes and essential oils), gold and precious stones to King Solomon. As far back as 2900 BC, the pharaohs and prominent Egyptians were buried in jars of perfumed oil after they died. Although perfumes, essential oils and spices were the provenance

---

16 Spikenard, also called nard, nardin, and muskroot, is a class of aromatic, amber-colored essential oil derived from *Nardostachys jatamansi*, a flowering plant of the Valerian family that grows in the Himalayan regions of Nepal, China and India.

of temples and the nobility, eventually their availability and use spread to the wealthy and then to the lower classes of the population.

Although the use of cosmetics, perfumes, essential oils and spices eventually must have extended throughout all levels of society, perfumes and oils were first used in "religious" ceremonies and for healing purposes (see later). In fact, they were central to cultic worship and witchcraft, with fragrant ointments being applied to statuary, and even to their attendants, to satisfy the "gods". It is possible that this practice of adorning statues and temple servants eventually led to personal use across society to enhance facial beauty and the body, and perhaps to conceal defects such as birthmarks and so forth. This is not quite the stretch it might appear to be because the pharaohs of Ancient Egypt were considered to be gods, and this "divinity" also was often the self-proclaimed right of Roman emperors. This deification possibly occurred with rulers in Ancient Greece but whether self-deification by rulers and potentates was part of the culture in Arabia, China, India and other ancient civilizations is unclear.

Because of the societal importance of unguents and various cosmetics for adornment, detailed recipes for formulations intended to remove or at least mask skin blemishes, wrinkling and signs of aging can be found in ancient papyri[17] from as long ago as the 16th Century BC. These ancient unguents contained fragrant oils and were used to anoint and perfume the skin but also appeared to have a symbolic significance in religious ceremonies. The unguents used for anointing the skin after bathing and for medicinal purposes apparently had a vegetable oil base, such as olive, almond, sesame or other oil, to which were added fixatives such as honey, milk, various salts and, notably, fragrant resins or aromatic flowers, i.e. essential oils. Washing the body and anointing it with oil was of great importance to the Ancient Egyptians, Romans and Greeks as well as the Israelites not only for hygienic reasons but also as an act of worship. The Bible and the Talmud make it

---

17   Papyrus (plural: papyri) is a material prepared in Ancient Egypt from the pithy stem of the papyrus plant, *Cyperus papyrus*, a wetland sedge. Papyrus was used in sheets throughout the ancient Mediterranean world to write or paint on and also for making rope, sandals, and boats. The term "papyrus" also refers to a document written on sheets of papyrus joined together side by side and rolled up into a scroll to become an early form of a book.

clear that the custom of washing the hands and feet was a venerable custom with major cultural and religious significance.

The use of unguents often had another and important purpose. In particular, facial cremes and lotions would protect the skin against sun damage as well as prevent severe dehydration in hot, dry climates. In addition, colored ointments applied around the eyes, what we now consider to be "eye makeup", prevented dryness and provided protection against inflammatory eye diseases, notably those transmitted by flies and other flying insects endemic to that region.

Essential Oils and Medicine

The known history of oleoresins and essential oils is intimately associated with both spiritual and medical overtones, particularly their usefulness in treating wounds and the healing of various pathological conditions. The venerable use of balsams (the aromatic resinous substances exuded by various trees and shrubs) as a base for certain fragrances and medical and cosmetic preparations as well as to treat wounds has several overtones. There might have been a conscious or perhaps an unconscious analogy between the healing powers of gums exuded by trees to heal injuries or wounds in their bark and the use of these gums for human wounds. Secondly, infected wounds smelled bad and the perfume or aroma of oleoresins not only eliminated the odor but helped the curative (skin repairing) process. In 300 BC, for example, Theophrastus[18] described the formula for a "perfume" containing burnt resin, cassia, cinnamon and myrrh that was intended to relieve wound inflammation. Thirdly, resins are one of the few products within nature that never degrade or decay, and the ancients might have considered that this characteristic was equally applicable to wounds and skin injuries.

The healing properties of essential oils and aromatics as well as those of herbs and plants are well established by numerous ancient documents, historical records and archeological material dating at least from the third millennium BC. These findings include mosaics, stone vessels, ovens, cooking-pots, clay jars and glass perfume flasks and they

---

18   Theophrastus, a native of Eresos in Lesbos, was a Greek philosopher, botanist and scientist who succeeded Aristotle as leader of the Peripatetics.

show how important body care and esthetics as well as medical treatments were in the lives of people throughout history. The Ptolemaic Temple of Horus, constructed between 237 BC and 57 BC on top of the remains of earlier temples at Edfu in Egypt, has many inscriptions on the walls of a perfume "laboratory" within the temple. Apparently, perfumes and scented ointments (unguents) were produced in such temple laboratories.

The ancient Greek writer Philostratus recorded that the priests of Asclepius, the "god" of medicine, apparently learned their healing arts through divination. Interestingly, the symbol of the Rod of Asclepius with a serpent coiled around the staff, was an ancient Greek emblem associated with medicine, and it is still used today by medical and dental professionals. It is also interesting and possibly no coincidence that a major temple of Asclepius was founded in the 4th Century BC on the island of Kos, the birthplace of Hippocrates.

Although medicinal concoctions such as salves, lotions and tinctures based on essential oils and perfumes have been known for literally thousands of years, the medicinal potency of those medications was probably somewhat limited. Although much of the modern usage of essential oils largely parallels that of the ancient past, it is likely that the oils and botanical extracts used over the millennia did not possess the purity or potency of what is available now. This lower biological efficacy of essential oil-based medicines in antiquity compared to present day oils may be due, at least in part, because of impurities and contaminants in the distillate, as previously mentioned.

In addition to the many references to oils and perfumes in the Bible and other spiritual texts, a large body of knowledge originated in the ancient Indian subcontinent. This knowledge was contained in writings known as the Vedas and which dated from about 2000 BC. Within roughly the same time period, writings from Ancient Egypt, notably Eber's Papyrus, which dates from about 1550 BC and believed to have been copied from other written work as old as 3400 BC, were also known. These venerable documents contained lists of medicinal plants and aromatics. This knowledge apparently was acquired by the Pythagorean philosopher Democrates and the Greek historian Heodotus, who both were thought to have visited Egypt around

425 BC, and the information they garnered then spread throughout Ancient Greece.

It is not clear when the medicinal properties of aromatic oils became established throughout Mesopotamia[19] but evidently, they had been used for this purpose over the millennia. Interestingly, Arabian frankincense and myrrh had far superior aromas than the other balsams which the Ancient Greeks and Egyptians customarily used as aromatic sources. In fact, the Ancient Egyptians imported huge amounts of Myrrh as early as 2500 B.C., although the proportion of these imports used for medical purposes is unknown. There are also numerous references in ancient papyri to resin-based wound salves and in 1370 B.C. Milkili, one of the lieutenants of the Egyptian pharaoh Amenophis IV (also known as Akhenaten), wrote to the pharaoh asking for supplies of myrrh to treat battle casualties.

The Ancient Greeks also used aromatic plants and bushes, principally the turpentine tree, for incense and to treat wounds. Herodotus (the 5th Century BC Greek historian and contemporary of Socrates) in his account of the Greco-Persian wars referred to the use of myrrh to tend the captain of a Greek trireme who suffered severe wounds in a naval battle around 480 BC. Hippocrates (460-370 BC), the "father" of organized medicine, recommended inhalation of aromatic vapor to treat disease and frequently prescribed myrrh to treat various conditions, including bacterial infections although it is unlikely that he would have used that term to describe infected wounds since bacteria *per se* were unknown at that time.

In the 3rd Century BC, the Greek botanist Theophrastus recommended a mixture of burned resin, cassia, cinnamon and myrrh for the relief of wound inflammation. It appears that the germicidal properties of oil of cinnamon were long recognized by ancient physicians. Expertise in wound healing was likely an essential skill for physicians in antiquity given the incessant wars being waged throughout the known world. Such wars and conflicts involved Egypt, Greece and

---

19 Mesopotamia is the historical region in Western Asia situated within the Tigris–Euphrates river system. In modern times, this region roughly corresponds to most of Iraq, Kuwait, parts of Northern Saudi Arabia, the eastern parts of Syria, Southeastern Turkey, and regions along the Turkish–Syrian and Iran–Iraq borders.

the Romans, as well as virtually every nation in the Middle East. Given the relatively poor hygiene in ancient days, it is no surprise that wound infections were endemic.

The Ancient Romans likewise were familiar with aromatic oils and archeological findings indicate that they used scented oils for a variety of medical purposes including massage therapy. Apparently, the Roman physician Celsus used a wine-myrrh lotion to treat bums around 100 AD. The Inner Cannon of China's Yellow Emperor, compiled 475-200 BC, also listed a wide variety of medicinal plants and aromatic oils although their precise identities are unknown.

In other words, essential oils, aromatics and perfumes were used extensively throughout the ancient world for spiritual, medicinal and other purposes for literally thousands of years. This situation changed with the fall of the Roman Empire.

Essential Oils in the Dark Ages and the Renaissance

From the start of the so-called Dark Ages[20], namely the early Middle Ages from about 460 to 1000 AD, the use of aromatic oils was strictly curtailed, and the Catholic Church even deemed bathing to be decadent if not sinful. At the same time, the Church also dismissed the holistic health-care and medical principles of Hippocrates, and healers who used essential oils, perfumes and herbs for their curative properties were often condemned for witchcraft and burned at the stake. It appears, however, that the art of essential oil extraction (i.e. distillation) and the use of essential oils in medicine and aromatherapy was continued in some secrecy by monks within their cloistered communities. This covert action apparently also applied to herbal medicine although it is possible, and highly likely, that aromatic oils and spices were in general use as air fresheners to offset the malodorous emanations from unwashed bodies.

---

20   The Dark Ages is the name given to the early Middle Ages from about 460 to 1000 AD. It refers to the period in western Europe between the fall of the Roman Empire and the high Middle Ages and during which Germanic tribes swept through Europe and North Africa, often attacking and destroying towns and settlements.

This situation continued until the advent of the Renaissance or what is known as the Age of Enlightenment (14th – 17th Centuries). It was during this period in history when personal hygiene and the use of essential oil and other plant-based remedies for medicine and to enhance the quality of life was once again deemed acceptable, if not necessary. Many physicians became adept at treating a wide variety of diseases and bacterial skin infections using herbal and plant-based (essential oil-containing) medicines, and probably prevented the spread of a great number of devastating diseases. This medicinal use of essential oils occurred without most physicians actually understanding the cause of the skin and other infections they were treating.

Knowledge of the ability of plant extracts to improve the course of wound healing became both widespread and acceptable from the Middle Ages onwards. Even Guido Majno, in his book[21] on wound healing in the Middle Ages, refers to a simple bacteriological study in which myrrh was tested against a selection of bacteria. It was found that myrrh dissolved readily in water and that it acts as a bacteriostatic agent against *Staphylococcus aureus* (a common wound bacterium and the cause of osteomyelitis, a frequently intractable bone infection) and other Gram-positive bacteria (see Appendix F). In other words, myrrh appears to exhibit comparable antibacterial effectiveness to penicillin and more modern antimicrobial drugs. By the 1600's, writings about herbal medicine and essential oils became widespread and most of the pharmacopoeias of England, Germany and France were referencing and promoting their use to treat a variety of illnesses over the next 200+ years.

During this period, large flower-growing districts in the south of France were supplying raw materials, presumably as essential oils extracted by enfleurage or distillation, to French perfumers. Although tuberculosis was endemic in many parts of Europe, workers who processed these flowers and herbs generally remained disease-free and this prompted some of the early laboratory-based (i.e. *in vitro*) studies of the anti-bacterial properties of essential oils. Interestingly, more recent scientific studies over the past few years have confirmed that certain essential oils, including citrus oil, citronellol, linalool and eucalyptol

---

21   Guido Majno: *The healing hand. Man and wound in the ancient world.* Harvard University Press, 1975.

oil, can inhibit the airborne transmission of tuberculosis by more than 90%.

Essential Oils and Modern Medicine

Although the effectiveness of essential oils (and their derivatives, perfumes) in wound healing and other health benefits had been recognized for literally thousands of years, it was only early in the 20ᵗʰ Century that modern medical science started to become seriously interested in them. In a serendipitous accident, a French cosmetic chemist, Rene-Maurice Gattefossé, severely burned his hands and arms in an accidental lab explosion in 1910. He extinguished the flames but as he described it, *"both my hands were covered with rapidly developing gas gangrene."* He treated his burns with lavender oil, reporting that *"just one rinse with lavender essence stopped the gasification of the tissue. This treatment was followed by profuse sweating and healing which began the next day."*

Although he previously had had no interest in natural healing methods, his astonishing burn experience led Gattefossé to evaluate the medical uses of essential oils by treating soldiers in military hospitals during World War I. He coined the term *"aromatherapie"* in 1920's-1930's to describe his treatment of disease and injuries using aromatic essential oils. Another Frenchman, Jean Valnet, a Parisian physician and army surgeon, began to use essential oils with great success as antiseptics and anti-microbials when treating war wounds during the Indochina war from 1948-1959. As the story goes, he was stationed in Indochina (now Vietnam) and treating wounded soldiers when his supply of antibiotics ran out. Out of desperation, he began to use essential oils on the injured men and was amazed at how well the essential oils fought infections, and he maintained that many lives were saved due to the use of essential oils. After the war, Valnet continued using essential oils in his private medical practice and in 1964 published the comprehensive textbook *The Practice of Aromatherapy*. This monograph earned Valnet global recognition and stimulated further scientific interest in the curative properties of essential oils.

In the 1980's the French physician, Daniel Pénoël, and his colleague, the biochemist Pierre Franchomme, investigated and catalogued the medical properties of over 270 essential oils. In 1990, they co-authored a reference book, *L'aromatherapie Exactement*, that listed the medicinal properties of essential oils. The book soon became the primary reference work for later research work on the medicinal properties of essential oils.

The medicinal use of essential oils over the millennia together with the almost explosive growth of the recent scientific literature in this area[22] clearly indicates the enormous potential of essential oils for the modern physician and healthcare provider. This is particularly true for those concerned with immediate (triage) treatment of wounds and similar injuries. The properties of myrrh, and presumably those of many other oleoresins, appear to make them very useful components of emergency medical kits and as well as adjunct anti-bacterial agents. In other words, because resins do not decay and they can be activated by dissolving in water, myrrh and similar ancient *perfumes* may be effective antibacterials without the limited shelf-life of modern antibiotics. Further, it is possible that their effectiveness may not be limited by the increasingly common, and very worrying, bacterial resistance found with modern antibiotic therapy.

The curative properties of essential oils and their role in modern medicine is expanded upon in Chapter 5. However, a note of caution must be sounded here. Some suppliers of essential oils make a variety of health-related and anti-bacterial claims for essential oils as well as for a variety of herbs and spices. None of these claims have been evaluated or are approved by the FDA and the use of essential oils for medicinal purposes should not replace proper medical treatment when indicated or displace personal judgment in treating any pathological condition. Of equal importance is that no claimed health benefits of essential oils should be understood to diagnose, treat, cure or prevent any disease.

---

22   J. A. von Fraunhofer: *Essential Oils. A Concise Guide*. CreateSpace/Amazon-Kindle (2017).

CHAPTER 5

ESSENTIAL OILS IN THE MODERN WORLD

T here was a major if not seismic shift in societal attitudes and behavior during the latter part of the 20th Century, a series of changes which now continue well into the 21st Century. Many of these changes are indicated in Table 5.1 and they have resulted in significant differences in human awareness and behavior.

Increased computer literacy
Greater health awareness and the effect of diet on health
Major shifts in societal and social mores
Heightened cynicism regarding politics and politicians
Lowered susceptibility to advertisements
A shift towards to alternative and complementary medicine
Greater consumption of "fast" foods
Greater prevalence of obesity and diabetes
Blurring of socio-economic boundaries
A major shift away from verbal to text messaging
Greater reliance on social media than on conventional news media
Lower prevalence of reading compared to TV viewing
Greater awareness of the benefits of regular exercise and relaxation

Table 5.1 Changes in Societal Attitudes in the 20th and 21st Centuries

Some of the most important of these societal changes are those in personal attitudes towards nutrition and healthcare but, at the same time, there is an increased consumption of "fast" or convenience foods with high salt and fat contents by many segments of the population. Bad diet and lack of exercise contribute to the modern near-epidemic of obesity, diabetes and cardio-vascular disease.

It is often said that there is little new under the sun, and this is particularly true for healthcare. Man has used different therapeutic approaches to treat a wide variety of ailments since the dawn of civilization. These traditional or folk remedies and treatments, Table 5.2, are commonly lumped together under the generic label of *complementary therapy and alternate medicine (CAM)* by Government agencies and organized medicine in developed countries. This somewhat dismissive attitude is particularly true when CAM therapies are used outside of their native cultures. On the other hand, most of these treatment modalities have been used since time immemorial (as discussed in Chapter 4). Even now in the 21st Century, the World Health Organization (WHO) indicates that up to 80% of the population in some Asian and African countries relies on traditional medicine for their primary health care.

Acupuncture	Islamic medicine
Ancient Persian medicine	Massage therapy
Aromatherapy	Muti Ifa
Ayurvedic medicine	Naturopathic medicine
Chiropractic	Shamanism
Essential oil therapy	Siddha medicine
Ethnomedicine	Traditional African Medicine
Folk medicine	Traditional Chinese medicine
Herbalism	Traditional Korean medicine
Holistic medicine	Unani
Homeopathy	Veganism

**Table 5.2 Traditional (folk) medicine and
alternate (complementary) therapies**

Many ancient practices such as massage therapy and aromatherapy that were dismissed or ignored by physicians and, latterly, modern medicine for hundreds of years have now been "re-discovered". This change in attitude and the reverting to age-old remedies and treatments has become increasingly popular because, quite simply, they have been found to be highly effective in treating so many different health conditions. This is particularly true for aromatherapy, massage therapy (especially when combined with aromatherapy) and the topical application of essential oils.

There is now an increasing trend in the oral use of essential oils to treat various digestive, respiratory and other systemic[23] health problems. Many medical practitioners and health professionals question the efficacy of the systemic health effects of essential oils, particularly their effectiveness in treating complex pathologies such as cancer and dementia/Alzheimer's disease. On the other hand, many of these oils have been certified as GRAS (Generally Recognized as Safe) by the FDA for oral consumption and there is a growing scientific literature on their therapeutic value in the treatment of a variety of conditions. For example, peppermint oil alone and in combination with caraway oil is reported to be effective for many gastric problems. Further, there are numerous anecdotal reports of aromatherapy with such essential oils as lavender, lemon balm and bergamot being effective for treating the symptoms of dementia, sleep disorders and anxiety as well as improving memory and cognitive function (see Chapters 7, 8 and 9).

Antimicrobial activity of essential oils

The therapeutic use of essential oils was practiced widely in the ancient world, as was the use of these oils for cosmetics, perfumes and personal care. In fact, many of the complementary and alternative medicine (CAM) therapies indicated in Table 5.2 either rely upon or involve the medicinal use of essential oils and other plant extracts and have done so for thousands of years. It is ironic that although essential oil-based healthcare was abandoned in the early centuries of the 1st millennium

---

23   The adjective *systemic* refers to the whole system (e.g. the entire body) rather just a single part.

AD, this practice now has become one of the new frontiers in pharmaceutical investigations.

Infections are caused by microscopic entities (collectively known as microbials) such as bacteria, viruses and fungi (see Appendix F). However, before discussing the therapeutic properties of essential oils and the growing body of scientific evidence and the plethora of anecdotal reports regarding this subject, the warning given at the end of Chapter 4 should be repeated here. In particular, no health-related claims (i.e. "drug" claims) made for essential oils or treatment modalities have been evaluated or approved by the FDA (U.S. Food and Drug Administration) and similar governing agencies in other countries. Further, the use of essential oils for medicinal purposes should not replace proper medical treatment when indicated or displace personal judgment in treating any pathological condition. Of equal importance is that none of these health benefit claims should be understood to diagnose, treat, cure or prevent any disease. Nevertheless, many suppliers of essential oils and a great many websites advance a variety of health-related claims for essential oils and many of these assertions are based on unsubstantiated anecdotal reports and lack scientific support or validation. This admonition applies to both humans and animals (see Chapter 10).

Bacteria

The word *bacteria* (the singular of which is bacterium) generally has a negative connotation because they are a cause of infections. This blanket disapproval is somewhat misleading because although some bacteria can be dangerous or injurious to health (i.e., they are *pathogenic*), a great many bacteria are beneficial, as is the case for the live cultures present in probiotics, yoghurt and other fermented dairy products. Not only that, non-pathogenic bacteria also are involved in such important processes as fermentation of grapes for wine and of hops in beer making as well as in various decomposition processes, e.g. sewage treatment.

Bacteria are microscopic single cell living organisms, hence they are termed *microbes* or *microbials*, and they are found everywhere in nature and especially in and on living organisms. The vast numbers of bacteria within the body are necessary for the overall health and viability of the human biosystem with over 400 different bacterial species existing in the gastro-intestinal tract (the gut), the skin, the vagina and the oral cavity. In fact, there are over 10^{14} bacterial cells (that is, 1,000,000,000,000,000 cells) in and on the body and their combined weight is about 3.3 lb. (1.5 kg) so that there are about 10 times as many bacterial cells in and on the body as the total number of cells that make up the human body. Bacteria and microbiology are discussed in greater detail in Appendix F (Bacteria and microbiological testing).

The bacteria within the gut (i.e., *enteric* bacteria) perform a variety of functions throughout the entire intestinal system, including being responsible for the bulk (70-80%) of the immune system. In general terms, a bacterium is "good" if it contributes to the health of its human host or at least is non-pathogenic whereas a bacterium is "bad" if it is pathogenic and can cause infections or if it is able to interfere with the proper functioning of "good" bacteria in the body. Augmenting and supporting gut bacteria as well as the immune system with prebiotics and probiotic bacteria is an important aspect of modern health care, and is discussed in Chapter 17 (Prebiotics, probiotics and gastric health).

On the other hand, a great many pathogenic (disease-causing) bacteria are found everywhere and they are the cause of serious, and sometimes fatal, diseases in man and animals. Unfortunately, once a bacterium enters the body, it can proliferate very rapidly, entering the bloodstream and organs to wreak havoc on the health of the "host". The immune system will mobilize to counter-act this bacterial invasion but if the extent of the invasion is so great that the immune system is overwhelmed, then additional counter measures, notably antibacterials must be administered. Compounding the problem is the fact that as bacteria proliferate, replicate and mutate with successive generations, each new generation can, and usually does, develop resistance to antibacterial medications. As a result, the efficacy of antibacterials (i.e., antibiotics) is reduced, often to the point that they no longer are effective, a depressingly common occurrence now.

After the fall of the Roman Empire (see Chapter 4) and until the advent of antibiotics, treating serious skin infections and wounds was difficult and often ineffective. Further, in many cases, the treatment caused as much if not more skin damage than the original wound, possibly because of impurities and adulterants in the medications being used. The same dilemma existed for systemic infections and millions of deaths occurred because the body and its immune system was unable to combat invading bacteria and fight off the effects of resistant pathogens.

This situation changed in the 1940's with the discovery of the first antibiotic, penicillin, together with subsequent technological developments that enabled its mass production. Since then, a plethora of antibiotics and anti-fungal agents have become available to successfully treat myriad pathological conditions. Unfortunately, due to overuse, overprescribing and often abuse of antibiotics over the past 50+ years together with changes (mutations) in the bacteria themselves, there has been a rampant proliferation of antibiotic-resistant bacteria. One example of this problem is *MRSA* or methicillin-resistant *Staph. aureus,* which is now almost impossible to treat except with the most powerful of antibiotics. Likewise, sudden outbreaks of severe intestinal problems due to antibiotic-resistant pathogens like *E. coli* are becoming increasingly common and tens of thousands of people are afflicted by "*Strep.* throat" every year. Increasingly sophisticated, and expensive, antimicrobials are now needed to treat such conditions.

Antibiotic-resistance of bacteria has made many serious systemic and skin infections increasingly difficult to treat and there is now a critical lack of antibiotics that can overcome recalcitrant bacterial infections. This distressing increase in antibiotic-resistant bacteria has led to a growing interest in alternative and "natural" approaches to treating skin infections and wounds as well as systemic pathologies, notably a return to CAM treatments and the use of essential oils. This therapeutic use of essential oils and other plant extracts is known as *phytomedicine* and has been a major component of traditional medical practices, as indicated above. There is also increasing interest in using phytomedicine to combat a variety of systemic infections using essential oils derived from less common botanical sources, e.g. those that grow naturally in locales like the Amazon basin.

Antibacterial properties of essential oils

The almost radical change in attitudes towards CAM modalities stems from the ground-breaking work of Gattefossé and Valnet in the 20th Century. These two men probably wrote the earliest modern monographs on the medical uses of essential oils, a practice they termed *aromatherapie*, which is "aromatherapy" in French, as discussed in Chapter 4. This use of the term *aromatherapy* is not the same as that referring to the aerial diffusion of aromatic/essential oils by diffusers (see Chapter 7, Aromatherapy). Prior to the work of Gattefossé and Valnet, numerous ancient writings by Egyptian, Greek and Roman authors were medical and pharmaceutical texts detailing the use of essential oils for treating a wide variety of conditions.

Since those days, there has been a growing body of scientific evidence regarding the antibacterial properties of certain essential oils. As previously stated in Chapter 4, the topical use of certain essential oils has long been advocated to promote wound healing and prevent infection through their antimicrobial activity. Most of the comments regarding the ability of essential oils to fight infections and, potentially, even cancer have been addressed in great detail elsewhere.[21]

The most familiar essential oils that are considered in many Online discussions and opinion pieces to have the highest antibacterial activity are indicated in Table 5.3, although many less-familiar if not uncommon essential oils are now known to have antibacterial properties, as discussed below.

Aniseed	Geranium	Nutmeg
Basil	Juniper	Orange
Camphor	Lavender	Oregano
Cedarwood	Lemon	Peppermint
Cinnamon	Lemongrass	Rosemary
Citronella	Lime	Sage
Clove	Linalool	Tea Tree Oil
Eucalyptus	Mint	Thyme
Frankincense	Myrrh	Wintergreen

Table 5.3 Essential oils claimed to have antibacterial activity.

Documented research studies and even quasi-scientific evaluations of the effectiveness of essential oil wound treatments have been lacking for millennia despite the many apocryphal and anecdotal claims regarding their use. This is no longer the case, and there has been a steady increase in the number of scientific studies of the antibacterial properties of essential oils reported in professional journals (i.e. the "literature") over many years. The antioxidant potential of essential oils has been confirmed in several scientific studies and literature reviews.[24]

The reports in the scientific and medical literature indicate that a great many essential oils are rich sources of biologically active (or *bioactive*) compounds, and their bioactivity against a diversity of pathogens has been confirmed. As a simple example, studies confirm that the myrrh is very effective in wound healing and it is unsurprising that myrrh was used as a field-dressing for battle wounds by the Ancient Greeks and, possibly, the Romans. Perhaps more interesting is that there is now evidence from animal studies that orally-administered myrrh may be helpful in gastric ulcer treatment. This assertion, however, is a *drug* claim and systemic use of myrrh has not been approved by the FDA or any other drug enforcement agency.

Overall, it has become increasingly apparent that traditional medicine and essential oils offer considerable promise in treating bacterial infections as well as many other pathological conditions. In addition to the familiar essential oils, several of the essential oils presently being studied for their antimicrobial (i.e. anti-bacterial) effects are extracted from plants that are less well-known and probably very unfamiliar to Westerners. The bioactivity of these "uncommon" essential oils has been the focus of many recent scientific studies evaluating their antimicrobial effects against bacteria, yeasts, filamentous fungi, and viruses. The findings of many of these *in vitro* or laboratory tests have been reviewed and discussed in a new book on essential oils (see Footnote 22). Without going into too many details as they are available elsewhere, it is interesting that modern science has confirmed the bioactivity of essential oils obtained from several plants that are listed in the well-established Chinese Pharmacopoeia. Although the original ver-

---

24   Amorati R, Foti MC, and Luca Valgimigli L. Antioxidant Activity of Essential Oils. J. Agric. Food Chem. (2013) 61: 10835–10847.

sion of this treatise is quite ancient, it has been revised and expanded for hundreds of years.

The essential oil derived from agarwood has been a component of Ayurvedic and Traditional Chinese medicine as well as in the folk medicine of many countries in South-East Asia, Bangladesh and Tibet. This essential oil has been used to treat joint pain, inflammatory-related ailments and diarrhea and, evidently, is thought to function well as a stimulant, sedative and cardioprotective agent. Scientific research has now proven that essential oils extracted from agarwood have complex chemistries. Further, clinical research (*in vitro* and some *in vivo)* studies indicate that they exhibit a wide range of actions including anti-microbial, anti-allergic, anti-inflammatory, anti-diabetic, anti-cancer, anti-oxidant and anti-ischemic activities. Similar findings are known for a great many other "traditional" essential oil medications that have been used for thousands of years.

Likewise, a rare plant species (*Thymus lanceolatus)* that grows wild in Algeria and Tunisia is the source of an essential oil which traditionally has been consumed as a beverage and used to both flavor and preserve meat and poultry. This essential oil has a complex chemistry, like most other essential oils, and recent scientific studies indicate it has very promising inhibitory activity not only against pathogenic bacteria but also against certain cancer cell lines in laboratory (*in vitro)* studies.

In the same region of the world, the essential oils from two species of the Salvia plant, which is indigenous to the Middle East, have traditionally been used in Lebanese folk medicine to treat microbial infections, cancer, urinary and pulmonary (lung and breathing) problems. Antimicrobial and anti-oxidative activity has also been found for essential oils extracted from other less-common plant species indigenous to the Mediterranean region and North Africa. This bioactivity has been endorsed by their inclusion in many traditional CAM therapies.

The Amazon basin is an incredible ecosystem with great biodiversity, and new species of animal and plant life are being discovered on an almost daily basis within the Amazonian jungles. It is unsurprising, therefore, that many botanical species indigenous to Amazonia would be the source of essential oils that possess bioactivity and antimicrobial activity. This antibacterial effectiveness has been confirmed by many recent research activities as has their cytotoxic (anti-cancer) activity. Many of these plants are discussed elsewhere (see Footnote 21).

Anti-cancer activity (Cytotoxicity)

The anti-cancer (cytotoxic) activity of essential oils is a highly contentious and emotionally charged subject because of the very nature and multi-faceted characteristics of the disease. Nevertheless, essential oils have been claimed to exhibit cytotoxicity properties for millennia and not all of these apocryphal and anecdotal reports should be dismissed out-of-hand.

Increasing numbers of scientific studies are now in progress into the anti-cancer effects of essential oils extracted from certain plants indigenous to the Middle East and elsewhere. In fact, reviews of the scientific literature from nearly 20 years ago and as recently as 2017 clearly show that bioactive phytochemicals in essential oils possess cytotoxic activity, suppressing tumor growth in laboratory (*in vitro*) studies and, interestingly, may also inhibit cholesterol synthesis in the body. In other words, modern clinical (*in vivo) and in vitro* research indicates that traditional (folk) medicinal approaches to treating cancer and many other diseases may have a sound and proven scientific basis.

What is also interesting is that the cytotoxic activity of essential oils extracted from cultivated plants is as good as that for essential oils extracted from wild-grown plants. For example, essential oils extracted from wild and cultivated *Salvia verbena* have comparable *in vitro* activity in inhibiting the growth of cancer cells and inducing apoptotic[25] cancer cell death.

It has already been stated that essential oils obtained from several plants found in the Amazon basin possess antibacterial activity, so it is perhaps unsurprising that cytotoxicity properties may also occur with essential oils extracted from plants growing in this incredibly diverse ecosystem. Research studies indicate that essential oils from many

---

25 *Apoptosis* is the term for the death of cells which occurs as a normal and controlled part of the growth or development an organism; this effect is also called *programmed cell death*. However, if a cell is sufficiently damaged (e.g. by a chemotherapeutic agent), it will respond by committing an orderly type of "suicide" or apoptosis, which stops it from causing any further problems.

Amazonian plants possess strong antibacterial activity and can exert significant *in vitro* activity against several tumor cell lines and *in vivo* antitumor activity in mice. In some cases, the antiproliferative activity (i.e., acting against the multiplication and spread of cancer cells) against an ovarian cancer tumor cell line was greater than that of the standard chemotherapeutic drug, doxorubicin.

Essential oils from plant species which are native to southern Europe, North Africa and Southwest Asia, namely the plant known as Nigella, Devil-in-a-Bush or Love-in-a-Mist, are potential chemotherapeutic and chemo-preventive anti-cancer agents. Likewise, another plant with the common names of Spicewood, Spicebush, and Benjamin bush that is native to Eastern Asia and the Eastern parts of North America is important in traditional Chinese medicine. Studies show that essential oils from this plant also exhibit cytotoxicity and antibacterial activity.

Another plant with the common name of Bitter Melon or Bitter Gourd is cultivated all over the world but notably in tropical areas of Asia, the Amazon region, East Africa, and the Caribbean. All parts of the plant, including the fruit, are consumed as food and will impart a slightly bitter flavor and taste when cooked with different vegetables in soups or sauces. Interestingly, Bitter Melon has been used for centuries in Ayurvedic (Indian traditional) medicine as a functional food to prevent and treat diabetes and associated complications. Now, recent research indicates that Bitter Melon has *in vitro* anti-tumor activity when tested against cell lines, inducing cell cycle arrest and apoptosis without affecting normal cell growth. The latter effect is in marked contrast to many chemotherapeutic agents used to treat cancer and which can wreak havoc on both healthy and cancerous cells.

One plant of major importance to modern anti-cancer therapy is the Madagascar periwinkle (*Catharanthus roseus*) which is the primary source of the chemotherapy drugs vinblastine and vincristine. These compounds are vinca alkaloids[26], originally derived from the periwinkle plant (*Vinca* rosea) and other vinca plants which are anti-mitotic

---

26 Alkaloids are a class of naturally occurring organic chemical compounds that mostly contain basic nitrogen atoms that have pronounced physiological actions on humans. They include many drugs such as morphine and quinine as well as poisons such as atropine and strychnine.

inhibitors and anti-microtubule agents.[27] In fact, vincristine, first iso-lated in 1961, is on the WHO's List of Essential Medicines, a list of the most effective and safe medicines needed in a health system. A tea made from the periwinkle apparently has been a traditional folk-rem-edy for diabetes.

Vinblastine is typically used with other medications to treat sev-eral types of cancer, including Hodgkin's lymphoma, non-small cell lung cancer, cancers of the bladder and the brain, melanomas and tes-ticular cancer. Likewise, vincristine (also known as leurocristine and marketed under various brand names including Oncovin) is a che-motherapy medication used with other agents in the treatment of a number of types of cancer. These include Hodgkin's lymphoma, neu-roblastomas, and small cell lung cancers as well as acute lymphocytic leukemia and acute myeloid leukemia. Although side-effects are found with both of these vinca alkaloids, they do not appear to elicit many of the adverse effects associated with several other (synthetic) chemother-apeutic agents. What is also interesting is that whereas the humble per-iwinkle plant produces vinblastine and vincristine naturally, synthesis of these two highly important therapeutic agents is presenting a major and almost insurmountable challenge to modern chemistry.

It is highly likely that there are considerably more anti-cancer agents to be found in numerous other plants. As modern medicine and pharmacology devote more time, energy and effort into investi-gating and evaluating traditional plant-based sources for medications, it is almost inevitable that many more life-saving therapeutics will be "discovered" by scientists the world over.

Probiotics

Another important example of the effectiveness of traditional or folk medicine is the regular and widespread consumption of probiotics and fermented foods like yoghurt for gastric health, to promote immune system health and to relieve a variety of conditions. Because many essential oils are bactericidal, there is growing interest in combining

---

27 *A mitotic inhibitor* is a drug that inhibits mitosis, or cell division. An anti-mi-crotubule agent disrupts microtubules, the structures that pull the chromosomes apart when cells divide.

medicinal plant extracts (i.e., essential oils) and probiotics to take advantage of their complementary antimicrobial effects with virtually no side effects.

This combined effect is apparently quite significant regarding antibiotic-resistant intestinal (enteric) pathogens. In other words, there appears to be a synergism[28] between essential oils and probiotics, the overall effect is that the combination may have a greater effect than that found with either of them acting alone. Probiotics, and prebiotics, are discussed in far greater detail in Chapter 17.

Final thoughts

It should be obvious from this chapter that modern science supports the curative properties of essential oils extracted from the indigenous plants used in traditional medicine. This increasing awareness of the benefits of CAM treatments is apparent from the multitude of *in vitro* (laboratory-based) and *in* vivo (animal and human) research reports in the scientific literature that now support and validate ancient beliefs and folk medical practices.

Scientific studies clearly show that the many terpenes, terpenoids and other compounds in essential oils have significant antimicrobial and anticancer activities. In addition, these bioactive constituents of essential oils appear to act synergistically, not only with each other but also with conventional chemotherapy and radiotherapy. Just how the anti-cancer (cytotoxic) effects of essential oils operate is unknown but could involve several different mechanisms. One possible role of essential oils could be to enhance or stimulate the immune system so that the body has a greater ability to fight off pathogens and cancer cells. Another factor is that because essential oils have complex chemical make-ups and a multitude of components, it is probable that there are synergistic effects both between these constituents and with those in other oils when blended together. This very complexity of natural essential oils not only accounts for their bioactivity but should also be

---

28 *Synergism* is the term applied to the interaction or cooperation of two or more organizations, substances, or other agents to produce a combined effect greater than the sum of their separate effects.

a warning against expecting synthetic essential oils to exhibit the same efficacy as pure, natural products.

The other facet of the antimicrobial activity of essential oils is that they may offer a solution to the modern and growing threat of increasing bacterial resistance to most antibiotics. Whether bacteria will develop a similar resistance to essential oils has yet to be determined but the fact that these oils have been used to treat skin and other pathologies with great effect for thousands of years suggests that loss of effectiveness against microbial organisms may not be a problem.

The reason for this apparent inability of microbial species to develop resistance to essential oils is that the botanical sources of the oils constantly undergo change from season to season. These natural changes in plant physiology occur in response to changes in the plant's environment, as discussed elsewhere in this book. Plants, almost by definition, are immovable and they respond in many ways to their changing environments in order to survive. Any climate and environmental changes for plants will obviously impact the chemical make-up, notably the minor components, of essential oils extracted from them. Consequently, the resulting changes in the proportions and concentrations of minor components will affect the anti-bacterial and cytotoxic activity of essential oils while neutralizing the tendency of bacteria to develop resistance to their clinical effectiveness.

Appreciation of such factors is certainly a contributing factor in the drive to characterize the therapeutic properties and clinical usefulness of essential oils. The rapid growth in the resistance of bacteria to antibiotics and the nearly empty pipeline of new antimicrobials stresses the importance of the anti-bacterial potential of essential oils. It is no wonder that modern medical science is "going back to basics" and re-examining traditional (CAM) treatments as well as devoting more attention to essential oils and their bactericidal and cytotoxic properties.

CHAPTER 6

TESTING AND ANALYZING ESSENTIAL OILS

When a bottle of Young Living essential oil carries a label that states that the contents are, for example, 100% pure, natural lavender oil, then there is an implied contract between vendor and purchaser that that is what is in the bottle. Merely stating what the bottle contents are, or what they should be, is not the same as being able to <u>prove</u> what is in the bottle. That is where QA/QC comes in. QA is quality assurance and QC is quality control and that is where Young Living devotes a great deal of time, trouble and expertise to ensure the quality and purity of its products. Achieving this high standard involves many factors, summarized in Table 6.1.

Highest quality botanical sources
Organically-farmed plants whenever possible
Meticulous harvesting and post-harvest handling of plants
Skilled distillation of the oils
High standards of cleanliness and purity throughout processing
Use of only contaminant-free and non-reactive processing equipment
Strict process control to prevent product mixing or contamination
Routine chemical testing of all products and production batches
State-of-the-art chemical test methods
Meticulous inventory, processing and laboratory records

Table 6.1 QA/QC requirements ensuring product purity

Most of these factors should be obvious and they are incorporated in Young Living's *Seed to Seal* philosophy. Central to the need to ensure product purity and absence of contamination, synthetics, pesticide/ herbicides or other unwanted species in the essential oils is the continuous physical and chemical analysis of all products using state-of-the-art analytical techniques and equipment.

Many different tests are performed to assure all staff and management of Young Living and, particularly, each member of the highest quality and purity of Young Living essential oils, oil blends and every other product. These testing regimens are performed throughout the entire production process and are shown schematically in Figure 6.1.

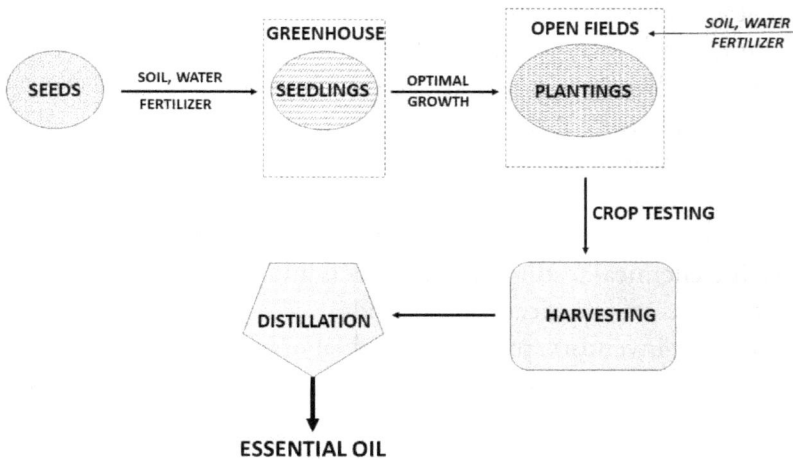

Figure 6.1 Schematic diagram of the Young Living production process

It should be noted that certain tests are performed even before plants are harvested and transported to the distillation operations. These tests on seedlings and plantings, and the times when they are performed, were outlined in Chapter 2.

Before going into details about the testing regimens adopted by Young Living, it might be useful to briefly discuss why superior companies direct considerable resources into quality assurance and quality control (QA/QC), research and development (R&D), as well as invest in a host of different analytical procedures and capabilities. QA/QC were discussed above regarding their importance in ensuring the quality and purity of Young Living products. A heavy investment in R&D is essential not only to ensure that essential oils are only extracted from premium plants by the best methods possible but also that the highest quality and innovative products are available to Young Living members. The importance of continuous R&D is discussed elsewhere in this book. Of almost equal importance to first rate QA/QC and R&D is the development of state-of-the-art testing and analytical capabilities.

Young Living, unlike many other companies, does not rely on third-party testing. There are two reasons for this. Relying on third-party testing can be fraught with risks because the data generated may not always be accurate and reliable. There can be many reasons why this unsatisfactory situation could arise with 3rd party testing. The chemists who perform the various analytical tests may rely on faulty, inadequate and sometimes inaccurate reference standards for the various test procedures (see later). Also, it is not uncommon for the personnel who perform third-party testing to lack appropriate skill levels, be careless or simply make mistakes in both the actual testing and the interpretation of the test data.... for some outside personnel, such testing is just "a job" not their livelihood. Secondly, Young Living's scientists have spent years developing very precise and carefully controlled test regimens as well as acquiring considerable expertise in performing the many testing and analytical procedures required to ensure the highest quality products. In other words, accuracy and precision for these in-house scientists is not just a requirement but an avocation. Consequently, Young Living has no need to rely on the potentially questionable findings and analytical work of third-party analyses. Nevertheless, Young Living does employ an extensive network of very skilled independent laboratories to perform highly specialized tests when such studies are deemed necessary.

Microbiological Studies

It should be mentioned that the overall production process incorporates a quarantine period of about 48 hours following distillation to ensure that the essential oil does not contain any microbial species such as bacteria, yeasts or fungi. By holding the essential oil in quarantine, there is ample time for microorganisms to multiply in the unlikely event that any such species are present within the distilled product. However, bacterial contamination of Young Living essential oils is highly unlikely, as discussed below.

The body contains billions of bacteria, many of which are "good" bacteria that are essential to the proper functioning of the human body but, as mentioned in Chapter 5, there are a considerable number of "bad" or pathogenic bacteria in nature. Good bacteria are the major component of probiotics (Chapter 17), and since the latter are important components of the health- and wellness-related products of Young Living, bacteriology and microbiology are covered in Appendix F. This

appendix discusses what bacteria are, what they do, how they are identified and classified and, to a degree, how they can be eliminated from
the body.

It is unlikely that Young Living essential oils contain microbial
matter for several reasons. First and foremost, the botanical plants that
are the source of essential oils predominantly are grown and harvested
following ecologically-sound farming principles. Second, the plants
are maintained in clean conditions and processing is undertaken as
soon as possible after harvesting to avoid any risk of contamination by
insects or other parasites. Thirdly, essential oils are extracted from their
botanical source by distillation, a process that involves the application
of heat under carefully controlled conditions. Generally, when microorganisms are exposed to heat, they undergo apoptosis or programmed
cell death due to this thermal effect. Finally, it is highly unlikely for
essential oils to contain bacteria or other microbes because these microscopic species must have an aqueous or water-containing environment
for them to survive and proliferate. Since, by definition, essential oils
are *oils*, they are water-free and therefore it is highly unlikely that they
will support microbial species. Nevertheless, Young Living does routinely perform certain microbiological tests to ensure that their products are contaminant-free.

Such testing involves placing a few drops of the essential oil on
a nutrient agar gel, which is very like gelatin or Jell-O, contained in a
glass or plastic container known as a Petri dish. After the Petri dish is
"plated", it is placed in an incubator so that any bacteria in the nutrient
gel from the oil can grow, an incubator being a closed cabinet that has
a temperature- and humidity-controlled environment.

Microbial growth is measured by the increase in the bacterial
population, either by measuring the increase in cell numbers (the
colony-forming units or CFUs) or the increase in the overall mass.
The basic method of evaluating bacterial growth is by cell or bacterial
colony counting with various methods being available for this. These
measuring methods include visual observation, flow and turbidity
measurements, biomass determinations and even nutrient uptake.

The results are commonly expressed as an MIT value, which is
the time that microorganisms are exposed to the test media and then
are visually inspected for viable microorganisms. If no growth occurs

within a specified time, then the sample material (the essential oil) is declared to be free of microbes and then can be evaluated for its other properties.

Bulk property testing

Many physical tests are routinely performed by Young Living on their essential oils and their many oil blends and specialized mixtures. These tests, Table 6.2, are performed to ensure that all products conform to the highest standards of purity and performance. Each test provides important information on the properties of the tested products before the essential oil is packaged and marketed. Another bulk property test, microbiological assessment, was discussed above and the importance and applications of refractometry were covered in Chapter 2.

Test	Characteristic
Clarity	Absence of sediment and inclusions.
Turbidity	Cloudiness/haziness due to presence of minute particles that are generally invisible to the naked eye.
Density (specific gravity)	Identifies pure substances and both characterizes and estimates the composition of mixtures. Indicates any dilution of the oil with other oils or solvents.
Polarimetry	Indicates that essential oil is pure and natural.
Refractometry	Measures the refractive index of a fluid.
Viscosity	Flow properties of fluids.

Table 6.2 Routine physical property tests

The types of physical tests and what these tests may, or may not, show is outlined in the right-hand column of Table 6.2. Obviously, any loss of clarity or the presence of turbidity within the essential oil indicates the presence of low levels of impurities or minute particulate foreign matter. Either of these conditions is unacceptable in a Young Living essential oil and, should they occur, steps would be taken immediately to remedy the situation or that particular batch of an essential oil would be scrapped.

Density or specific gravity measurements are routinely performed on essential oils because it is almost a "quick and dirty" guide to oil purity as well as a reliable indication of the composition of a mixture or blend of essential oils. In other words, density measurements are an immediate and reliable guide to any dilution or adulteration of an essential oil through the addition of carrier oils like coconut oil or diluents such as solvents. This is an important consideration since many so-called pure or all-natural essential oils are commercially available but, regardless of the bottle label, these oils may not be either pure or all-natural.

Polarimetry (see Appendix A), a measurement of the rotation of polarized light by a liquid, is performed to ensure that an essential oil is 100% pure and natural. Changes in the rotation of the light passing through an essential oil in a polarimeter will indicate lack of purity and/or that the oil is not a natural product. As a QA/QC tool, polarimetry will immediately detect the presence of diluents in "100% pure" oils which can then be identified by chemical analysis. It will also readily distinguish between synthetic oils and those that are derived from natural botanical sources.

The viscosity or flow properties of an essential oil is not, in itself, a very important characteristic of a pure essential oil. However, flow properties can be a consideration with oil blends that are intended for use in massage therapy and, perhaps, also with topical aromatherapy. Ideally, an essential oil blend intended to be used in massage therapy should flow easily but not be so runny that it will flow too quickly over the skin and slip off or away from the body like water. Likewise, the oil blend should not be so viscous that it does not flow well or resists smoothing across the target area; in other words, oil blends that are as viscous as, say, honey would be unacceptable to most massage therapists.

In the unlikely event that any batch of an essential oil or a blend does not satisfy the rigorous test criteria established by the QA/QC team at Young Living, then that particular batch is scrapped because it does not meet the requisite standards.

Many of the tests indicated in Table 6.2 are cited in National and International standards. ISO (International Organization for Standardization) and ASTM International (American Society for Testing of Materials) both have voluntary consensus technical standards for essential oils. Further, the ISO has adopted the AFNOR (Association Française de Normalisation) standards for essential oils. At present, no company certifies its essential oils although ethical corporations such as Young Living do use these guidelines as well as their own internal standards for testing their products. This company testing policy ensures that the oils and blends they create preserve the properties and integrity of their essential oils, supporting their effects on the body and emotional wellbeing. In fact, Young Living regularly sends samples of its oils to independent laboratories in France for testing against *AFNOR/ISO* standards.

Chemical tests

It has been stated previously in this book that essential oils are multi-component mixtures with complex chemistries. Further, essential oils can contain up to 100 separate components, many of which are present in relatively small amounts. This large number of compounds presents a major challenge to QA/QC and analytical chemists. The many minor components in an oil contribute to the properties of that oil, particularly such important characteristics as its aroma and bioactivity. Not only that, the constituents of the oil will clearly indicate its botanical source, notably where it was grown, when and how it was harvested and the presence or absence of adulterants, herbicides, pesticides and pollutants. It will also indicate which minor ingredients are naturally present in that oil, and those that may have been accreted or accumulated during any stage of the overall production process.

Detailed chemical analysis of essential oils is important because it is not uncommon for cries of fake horror to be uttered by uninformed people and even by some of Young Living's competitors regarding very minor amounts of certain naturally occurring components that are always present in essential oils. There are many classic examples of this phenomenon, one of which is the naturally occurring presence of 0.04% (i.e., 400 ppm or 400 parts per million) of toluene in frankincense. That minute presence is not injurious to health and since frankincense has been a staple of folk medicine and incense for thousands of years, there is no reason to ever expect it to cause problems. It is also interesting that if such minor components are <u>not</u> present in an essential oil, then that missing component is a very clear if not a give-away indication that the bottled product in question is not pure, natural or what it is purported to be from the label.

Another example of mock horror stories regarding minor ingredients, in a completely different area, is the naturally occurring presence of 1 ppm fluoride in tap (drinking or potable) water. Since this amount equates to about ½ a restaurant packet of sugar dissolved in a gallon of water, it is hard to rationalize that it could possibly relate to assertions that fluoride is a rat poison and should not be present in drinking water. In fact, meticulous medical and dental studies have shown that the only difference between the populations of matched towns with naturally fluoridated water and those with fluoride-free water is the markedly lower rate of dental decay (cavities) when fluoride is present.

Clearly, identifying the components and their relative amounts or concentrations in any given essential oil provides the biological equivalent of a "fingerprint" of that oil. Also, the presence or absence of certain minor ingredients in an essential oil is a very accurate indicator of whether that oil is natural or synthetic, see Appendices B, C, D and E. At the same time, any diminution in the relative concentrations of the diverse components in a sample of an essential oil will clearly indicate adulteration of that oil. Likewise, precise chemical analyses will show if there has been mixing of oils from plants grown and harvested in different locales, or even different countries. This is because, as noted in Chapter 2, the soil, climate, ground water and harvesting all affect the composition of essential oils extracted from botanical sources grown in different regions.

Unfortunately, merely stating that chemical analyses are performed on essential oils does not reflect the difficulty, expertise and highly sophisticated equipment required to perform such testing. The most important testing regimens for essential oils are Fourier-Transform Infrared Spectroscopy (FTIR), chromatography, mass spectrometry and GC-MS (gas chromatography-mass spectrometry). Whereas most readers of this book have come across these chemical analysis techniques in books, online articles and, particularly, several popular television dramas, few may know anything about them. This is unsurprising because they all involve a lot of heavy-duty and arcane science that is difficult to understand, even for many scientists. For the interested reader, Appendices B-E of this book provide further information on what these analytical methods comprise and the information they provide.

Infra-red Spectroscopy

Infrared spectroscopy is an analytical method that utilizes the interaction of infrared (IR) light with a molecule. This interaction of the molecule with the incident IR light can be analyzed in three ways, namely measuring the absorption of the incident light by the oil being tested, measuring emission of IR light after absorption by the oil or determining the reflection of the incident IR light by the tested oil. The main use of this technique is in organic and inorganic chemistry to determine functional groups in the molecules of the compound or mixture being tested. The scientific principles behind this technique are discussed in Appendix B.

The IR spectrum of a molecule or mixture has two main regions, one extending over the wavenumber region of 4000-1500 cm^{-1}, and a second region, extending from 1500 down to 500 cm^{-1}, the latter region being known as the fingerprint region. The individual peaks in the fingerprint region are very important because, like human fingerprints, they are unique to the individual molecule (compound) under examination.

However, whereas IR spectroscopy will identify different molecules, in general it is not able to readily distinguish between pure, natural essential oils and synthetic oils that are nominally the same, i.e. that have the same major component. This difficulty can be seen by comparing Figure 6.2, the IR spectrum of 100% pure wintergreen oil, with the IR spectrum of a synthetic wintergreen oil, Figure 6.3, the two spectra being nearly identical.

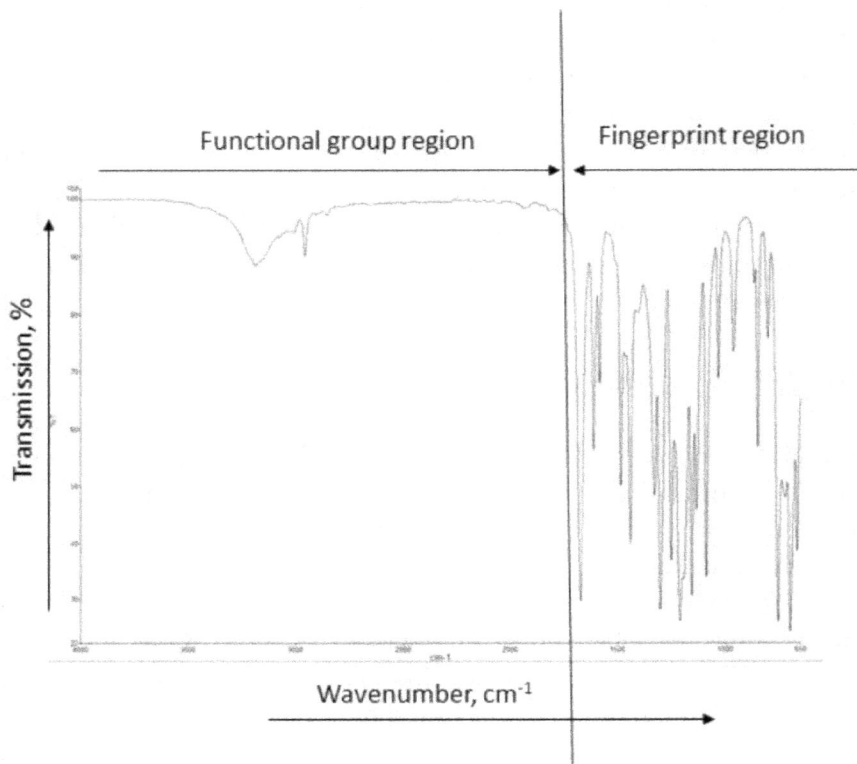

Figure 6.2 IR spectrum of 100% pure, natural wintergreen oil [Courtesy of Young Living]

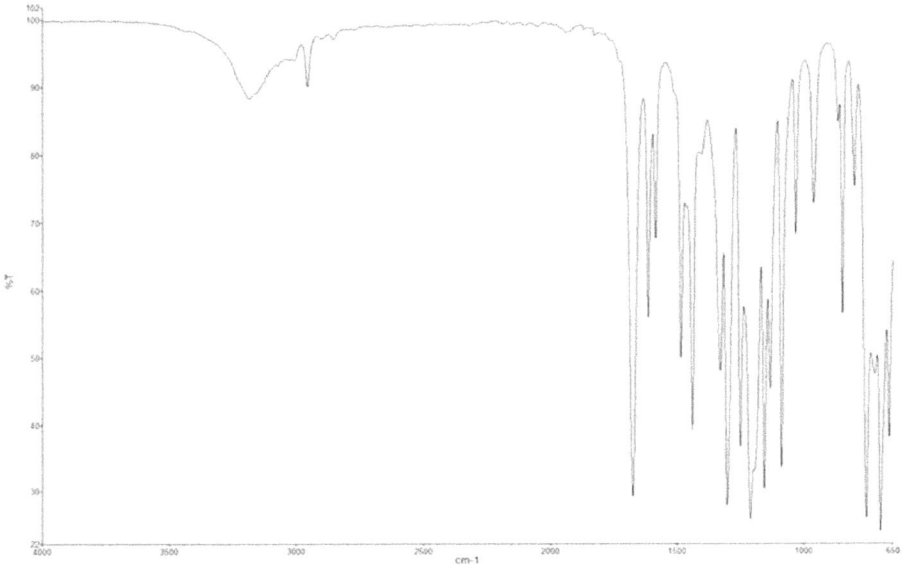

**Figure 6.3 IR spectrum of synthetic wintergreen
oil [Courtesy of Young Living]**

In order to distinguish between natural and synthetic essential oils, and to fully characterize them, chemists must use a different analytical technique. The most common approach to addressing this problem is GC-MS or gas chromatography-mass spectrometry.

Gas Chromatography (GC-MS) Analyses

GC-MS is routinely used by Young Living as part of its QA/QC protocols and the instrumentation employed is state-of-the-art. In fact, a variety of instruments are available that permit "customization" of each analysis. For example, different types of columns are used in the gas chromatography (GC) part of the GC-MS system. Because columns of different dimensions and specialized stationary phases are used, very precise separation of the components in the essential oils is performed on a routine basis. The mass spectrometry (MS) part of the instrumentation is equally state-of-the-art and innovative. The instruments and their operating software in the analytical test laboratories allow selected-ion-monitoring (SIM) and full mass/charge (m/z) scans, see Appendices C, D and E. The instrumentation and software also permit adjusting the measurement sensitivity across selected m/z ranges so that specific components can be detected and measured in the sample of essential oil being tested.

The analytical capabilities and versatility of GC-MS is shown by the following GC-MS chromatograms for synthetic and 100% natural wintergreen oils.

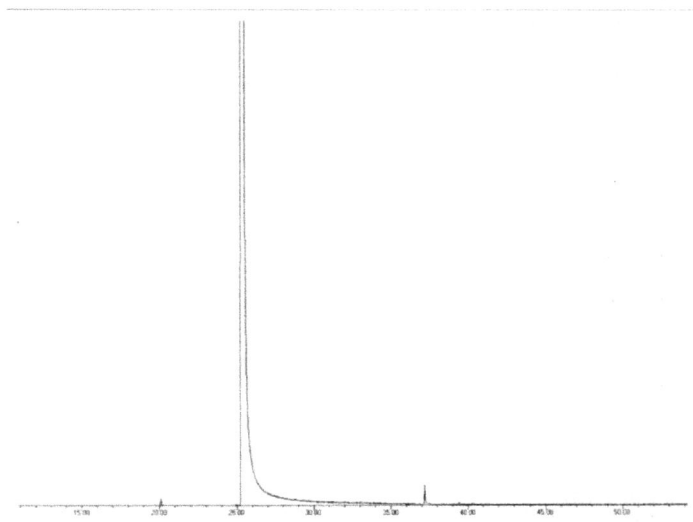

Figure 6.4 GC-MS chromatogram of synthetic wintergreen oil [Courtesy of Young Living]

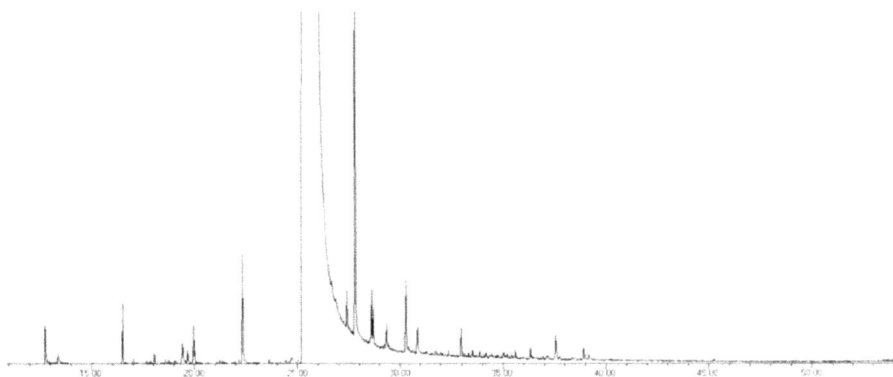

**Figure 6.5 GC-MS chromatogram of 100% natural
wintergreen oil [Courtesy of Young Living]**

It is immediately apparent by comparing Figures 6.4 and 6.5 that
the GC-MS chromatogram of synthetic wintergreen oil has only three
peaks or lines whereas the chromatogram for the genuine (100% pure
and natural) wintergreen oil has many more peaks. The smaller peaks
or lines indicate the minor components in the pure, natural essential
oil and are a "virtual fingerprint" of the natural product. It is these
minor components that account for the properties and characteristics
of natural products.

In order to correctly interpret the chromatograms of unknown
samples produced by GC-MS, pure and unambiguous standards must
be used to calibrate the system so that the sample spectrum can be elu-
cidated accurately. The chromatograms for both known and unidenti-
fied essential oil samples are compared with the data in large libraries
of mass spectrograms that are available. One such mass spectral library,
NIST 17, is available from the National Institute of Standards and
Technology (NIST), Gaithersburg, MD. This library is a fully evaluated collection of mass spectra with chemical and GC data together
with search software to identify unknown spectra. It is a compilation of
a more than a three decade-long comprehensive evaluation and expan-
sion of the world's most widely used mass spectral reference library by a

team of experienced mass spectrometrists at NIST This comprehensive library is augmented by Young Living's own internally-developed MS library that is specific to essential oils and their often-extensive range of components. The availability of these libraries facilitates identification and quantification of essential oils although interpretation of GC-MS data requires experience and skill on the part of the chemists performing these analyses.

Young Living maintains careful records of the physical and chemical (analytical) tests performed on essential oils so that there is a continuous record of the composition of every Young Living product that is marketed. This is because although there will inevitably be some variations between the chromatograms (and the other analytical data) for different batches of an essential oil, there should be a general consistency from batch to batch. The variations in composition and/or relative amounts of minor ingredients that do occur are to be expected because the botanical source of that oil is always a seasonal crop. As indicated in Chapter 2, small changes in the local climate, soil quality, ground water and so forth during the growing seasons will be reflected by small variations in individual crops. These differences cause small changes in the plants each year and, therefore, the extracted essential oils will vary from year to year. In other words, when identical GC-MS data are found for different batches of an essential oil, then this is a clear sign that something is not right.

Essential Oils and Their Properties

The bioactivity of essential oils was discussed in Chapters 4 and 5. Most, but not all, of these effects may be ascribed to the principal components, i.e. those present at the highest relative concentrations. The minor components or *conjoiners* in an essential oil, see Figure 6.5 above for example, are what give the oil its characteristic properties and often are the source of the differences between nominally the same essential oil supplied by different companies. In some cases, the presence of certain minor components in an impure or diluted essential oil can often be the cause of adverse effects such as allergic reactions or other consequences that have been found with the products of some companies. On the other hand, minor components in pure, natural oils, even at relatively low concentrations, can have remarkably beneficial effects on, as well as contributing to, the oil's bioactivity. In fact, many of these minor ingredients can act synergistically with each other and with the principal component so that their combined effects are markedly greater than those ascribable to each ingredient or component acting alone. As a result, it is not unusual that minor components in an essential oil can often have a disproportionately large effect on the overall properties of that oil. It is for this reason that synthetic oils, which do not contain these minor components, are unable to provide many if not most of the health benefits of 100% pure and natural oils.

Clearly, careful analysis and characterization of all essential oils is necessary to ensure that customers have available to them products of the highest quality and absolute purity. This objective is exemplified by the *From the Ground Up* philosophy of Young Living.

CHAPTER 7

AROMATHERAPY

Aromatherapy is that form of alternative or complementary medicine which uses the natural oils extracted from flowers, bark, stems, leaves, roots or other parts of a plant (i.e., the essential oils) to enhance physical and psychological well-being. The underlying basis for aromatherapy is that the inhaled aroma from these essential oils stimulates brain function. Essential oils can also be absorbed through the skin and when they travel through the bloodstream to be distributed throughout the body, they can promote whole-body healing, as in massage therapy (Chapter 9).

Using aromatherapy to address a variety of mental and physical problems is gaining momentum world-wide and its applications include pain relief, mood enhancement, relaxation and increased cognitive function. Overall, patients and users find that aromatherapy enhances the quality of life (QOL) by improving their psychological, spiritual and physical well-being. Anecdotal, apocryphal and now, increasingly, clinical studies indicate that aromatherapy can help with an array of symptoms and conditions, notably in mood enhancement, for stress relief and to offset anxiety and depression as well as to limit pain. It is also used to improve cognitive function and, remarkably, to enhance the mental processes of thinking, reasoning, remembering and imagining.

Aromatherapy has been in active use for thousands of years. Interestingly, Assyrian medical texts from Ancient Iraq recommend inhaling the fumes from burning cannabis to dispel sorrow or grief. As they say, there is nothing new under the sun.

Such noted advocates of the antibacterial activity of essential oils, namely Gattefossé[29] and Valnet[30], referred to this particular use of essential oils as "aromatherapie" (the French word for aromatherapy). Other workers have used a similar nomenclature in reporting their research studies with essential oils. In the context of this book, however, "aromatherapy" refers only to the effects of inhalation of essential oils.

THE SENSE of SMELL

Few people are immune to the effect of aromas and pleasant smells. Most delight in smelling a rose and even people who don't drink coffee will admit to liking the aroma of fresh-ground coffee beans. Aromas have an evocative, almost subliminal effect on the mind, and the conjuring up of memories by different smells is very common.

The importance of the olfactory system, i.e., our sense of smell, known by the scientific term *osmesis*, is underlined by the fact that one of the main sensory inputs to the brain is smell. The loss of the sense of smell can be partial (*hyposmia*) or complete (*anosmia*), and may be temporary or permanent, depending on the cause. *Congenital anosmia* (inability to smell or lacking a sense of smell from birth) is uncommon although some people may be anosmic or unable to smell a particular *odor* or aroma (a condition known as *specific anosmia*). Likewise, *hyposmia*, a decreased ability to *smell anything, is not uncommon, particularly when suffering from a cold, influenza or blocked sinuses.*

What is interesting about the sense of smell is that unlike other senses such as sight and hearing, odors are extremely difficult to measure quantitatively. Consequently, odors (aromas or smells) are clas-

29   René-Maurice Gattefossé, French chemist and perfumer, who used the term *aromatherapie* (French for aromatherapy) in 1920s and 1930s when referring to the treatment of disease and injury using aromatic essential oils. [Tisserand, RB. Gattefossé's Aromatherapy. C. W. Daniel Co. Ltd., Saffron Walden, U.K. (1995)]

30   Jean Valnet, French physician, who documented the use of essential oils for medical purposes, notably the treatment of skin infections and wounds. [Valnet, J. The Practice of Aromatherapy. Healing Arts Press, Randolph, VT (1990)]

sified subjectively and usually as metaphors, e.g. an odor may be described as fruity, smoky, like vanilla or chocolate, and so forth. The difficulty in classifying aromas has always presented a challenge to perfumers although progress is being made with the development of "smell" wheels that are used to characterize odors.

The important connection between aromas and the brain has been recognized since early times. There are, for example, numerous references to perfumes in the bible (e.g. Ecclesiastes 7:1) and the story in the Gospel of Mark (Mark 14:3-5) of the woman who entered the home of Simon and anointed the head of Jesus with perfume made from essence of nard (lavender oil).

Literature also has many references to perfumes. One example is Achilles perfuming the body of Patroklos with nard (lavender) oil[31] while Shakespeare, a great advocate of perfumes, wrote:

All the perfumes of Arabia will not sweeten this little hand[32]; and
So perfumed that the winds were love-sick[33]

and not even the great John Milton was immune to commenting on perfumes:

Sabean odors from the spicy shore of Araby the blest[34]

In other words, not only have perfumes and their source, essential oils, been regarded as very valuable since ancient times but the pleasing and calming effects of perfumes on human emotions have been recognized since Biblical times[35], and almost certainly before then. What is extraordinary is that scientific studies using electroencephalograms (EEC) patterns (i.e., instruments used to study brain waves) and other advanced brain imaging techniques have shown that odors and aromas

---

31   Homer's *Iliad* (Book 18)

32   Macbeth V.i

33   Antony and Cleopatra II.ii

34   Paradise Lost IV. 162-163 (Note that *Sabean* here refers to the language spoken by the *Sabeans* who lived in the land of Sheba, an area that is now Yemen).

35   2 Corinthians 2: 14 and 2: 16

can produce specific effects on human neuropsychological and autonomic[36] functions. In particular, clinical research studies show that aromas can have emotional effects such as influencing mood, perceived health, and arousal. So, modern science has confirmed centuries' worth of anecdotal and apocryphal comments that the aromas of essential oils and perfumes influence the mind and its emotions. Further, the indications are that the effect of essential oils on brainwaves and their ability to modify behavior most probably occurs via signals from the olfactory system transmitted to the brain.

It should be obvious from this that aromatherapy not only may have significant mental and spiritual benefits, but that the efficacy of these effects is now supported by scientific studies.

AROMATHERAPY

The basis for aromatherapy is that the inhaled vaporized matter (the aroma) from essential oils is thought to stimulate brain function, a perception supported by scientific evidence. Not only that, because essential oils also can be absorbed through the skin, topical application of EOs is believed to promote whole-body healing because they are transported throughout the body by means of the bloodstream.

The most common methods of utilizing aromatherapy are:

- Aerial diffusion for environmental fragrancing and purification,
- Topical application to the skin or clothing providing direct inhalation for respiratory disinfection, decongestion and stimulation of expectoration as well as psychological effects,
- Adding essential oils to warm bath water, and
- Topical application in massaging, bathing, compresses and skin care.

Of these, the most convenient approach is to evaporate the essential oils into the air by means of a diffuser, Figure 7.1.

---

36   The term *autonomic* refers to involuntary or unconscious actions/reactions and relates to the autonomic nervous system.

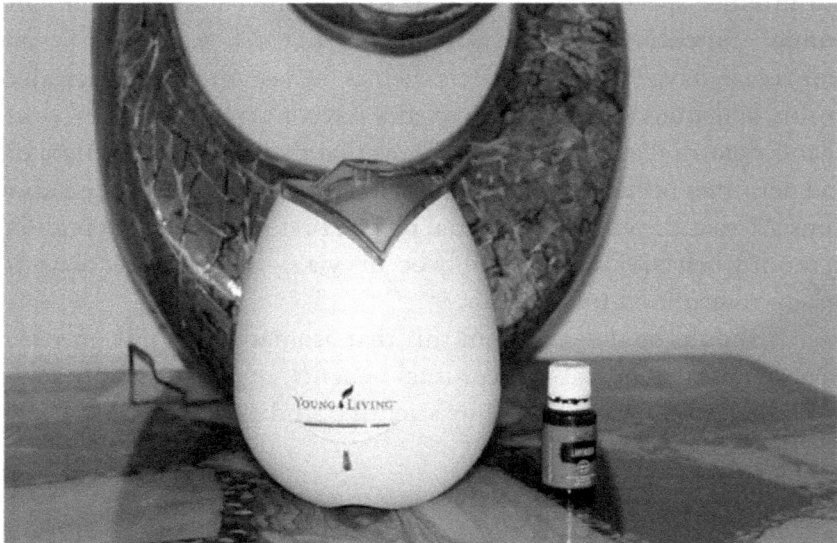

Figure 7.1 Aerial diffuser (nebulizer) of essential oils

Essential oils recommended for aromatherapy are indicated in Table 7.1. Note that the associated comments to that table have not been evaluated by the FDA and none of these products are intended to diagnose, treat, cure or prevent any disease.

Although most essential oils can be used in diffusers for aromatherapy, the table has notations indicating which oils are advocated for certain properties or applications:

> *: calming or relaxation properties
> #: spiritual uplifting and inspiration
> ^: energizing effects
> %: to improve concentration.

Angelica*	Goldenrod*	Orange *%
Basil*	Grapefruit^	Palmarosa*
Bergamot*#	Helichrysum%	Palo Santo#
Black pepper^	Hinoki#	Patchouli*
Cardamom#	Hong Kuai#%	Peppermint*
Carrot seed*	Hyssop%	Petitgrain^
Cedarwood*	Idaho balsam fir*	Pine*
Celery seed*	Idaho blue spruce*	Ravintsara#
Cinnamon bark^	Jade lemon^	Rose*#
Cistus*#	Jasmine*	Rosemary#
Clary sage*	Juniper*	Royal Hawaiian
Coriander*#	Lavender*#	sandalwood#%
Cypress*	Laurus Nobilis^	Sacred frankincense#%
Dill*	Ledum^	Sage*%
Eucalyptus blue*^	Lemon myrtle^	Spearmint*#
Eucalyptus Radiata^	Lime^	Tangerine^
Fennel#	Mastrante*	Taragon*
Frankincense*#	Melissa#^	Thyme%
Galbanum^	Myrrh#	Valerian*
Geranium*#	Myrtle^	Vetiver*
German chamomile*	Neroli^	Wintergreen#%
Ginger^	Northern Lights black spruce#%	Xiang Mao#
	Nutmeg^	Ylang ylang*

Table 7.1 Aromatherapy Oils

The usual application rate is to add 8-12 drops of essential oil to ½ cup (4 oz.) of distilled water in a diffuser such as the one shown in Figure 7.1 Certain essential oil producers such as Young Living also formulate oil blends to achieve specific aromatherapy effects by aerial diffusion and/or topical application. They also compound essential oil blends for massage therapy (see Chapter 9 and the Young Living Product Guide). Even a brief review of the ingredients that comprise these blends will indicate that these blends are complex mixtures. Further, these blends have been formulated to achieve certain, often quite specific, effects.

As already mentioned, essential oils may also be applied to the skin or clothing so that their aroma is directly released to the patient. A popular and well-established application of this principle is Vicks VapoRub®, a gel product containing a combination of peppermint, eucalyptus, and camphor essential oils. This classic aromatic ointment is a topical cough medicine with medicated vapors that works quickly to relieve coughs and nasal congestion for children and adults.

AROMATHERAPY and HOT FLASHES

Hot flashes, which the medical profession calls *menopause flushing*, are generally considered to be the primary symptom of menopause. Millions of women are affected by hot flashes and while they do not pose any direct danger to health, they certainly decrease the quality of life (QOL). Unfortunately, anything that adversely affects QOL can have major effects on mental and physical health.

The causes of hot flashes are not wholly understood but they are thought to be caused by a lack of the hormone, estrogen. Lowered levels of estrogen apparently cause the brain to detect too much body heat and the body responds by releasing hormones that increase the heart rate and pump more blood. This, in turn, causes blood vessels in the skin to dilate. The consequence of this cascade of reactions is that the body switches to its normal cooling method, namely sweating. The net result is menopausal hot flashes.

Hot flashes also may result from stress-released hormones like adrenaline, eating hot and spicy foods, caffeinated beverages, alcohol and smoking. Hot flashes also may be exacerbated by being overweight or obese. Certainly, a healthy diet, losing weight, not smoking, regular exercise and practicing relaxation can all help with hot flashes.

The most effective medical treatment for relieving the discomfort of hot flashes is to take estrogen, often in combination with other hormones.... what is known as hormone replacement therapy or HRT.

Unfortunately, there are risks involved with HRT, including heart disease, stroke, breast cancer and other serious conditions. Links have also been reported between HRT and dementia, Alzheimer's disease and other effects on the brain. Alternative medications are available for treating hot flashes but, as with any medication, there are always associated side-effects. Understandably, a great many women prefer not to undergo HRT or take medications for their hot flashes.

Many women resort to dietary supplements to relieve menopause symptoms including plant estrogens, black cohosh, ginseng, Dong quai and Vitamin E. However, studies indicate that these various treatments have mixed results or are ineffective, and some may even interact with prescription medications.

The good news is that a recent clinical study has found that the use of lavender oil aromatherapy reduced menopausal hot flashes, helped restore previously disturbed sleep patterns and induced feelings of calmness and peace of mind. The study validated long-held anecdotal and apocryphal comments regarding the benefits of aromatherapy for hot flash sufferers. In other words, this simple, safe and noninvasive approach has been found to be an effective method for menopausal women to deal with hot flashes as well as markedly improving QOL.

AROMATHERAPY and THE MIND

It is interesting that despite man being on the earth for thousands of years and despite most of us tending to agree with the old adage that "there is nothing new under the sun", we seem to regard mental illness as a "modern affliction". In fact, mental illness has been around since the dawn of civilization. This is not surprising since the human brain has not really changed or developed that much since Neanderthal man although the knowledge base in almost every field has expanded almost beyond belief in the intervening millennia. So, it is not remarkable that people have been using essential oils to heal the mind and body for centuries because then, as now, the positive effects of essential oils and aromatherapy on us are astounding. The scent of mint, for example, may make you feel more alert because it stimulates a nerve that allows one to perceive irritation and pain, and be aware that pain is no longer felt.

Aromatherapy is increasingly popular with the general public and has made its way into the offices of health care providers as well as spas and fitness centers. Nevertheless, there are few clear indications for the therapeutic use of aromatherapy. This is because it is very difficult to scientifically evaluate the clinical effectiveness of inhaled essential oils. Since patients enrolled in a clinical trial can smell the aroma, they are immediately aware that they are inhaling an aromatic and potentially curative substance. As a result, the trial participants are likely to expect a beneficial effect and will respond affirmatively when asked about their reactions by the scientists conducting the test regardless of whether the anticipated benefits really exist. This is known as the Hawthorne effect.[37] Nevertheless, the conclusions of most health care workers using aromatherapy as well as the reported findings of the limited number of controlled scientific studies all indicate that aromatherapy can have a beneficial effect in relieving anxiety and depression as well as reducing post-operative nausea and vomiting. In addition to these calming effects, specially blended essential oils mixtures can stimulate the mind and the spirit as well as have an uplifting and an enlightening influence on those exposed to the aromas.

So, clinical trials continue world-wide to validate (or dismiss) the health benefit claims of aromatherapy, but the consensus is that aromatherapy can be effective in many situations. An example of the beneficial effects of aromatherapy is in the treatment of individuals in emotional distress. Affected patients are often treated with psychotherapeutic agents but there is increasing evidence that aromatherapy is a safe, effective and convenient adjunct for the alleviation and treatment of emotional distress. In fact, there is growing scientific evidence that sufferers with PTSD and many other depressive conditions often find that aromatherapy can help them to manage their symptoms. Once the safe administration of essential oils is understood and the oils which provide the best results are identified, then many sufferers find that aromatherapy offers relief from even the most severe depressive conditions, including PTSD. The application and effectiveness of aroma-

---

37 *The Hawthorne effect* (also known as the observer effect) is a type of reaction in which individuals modify or improve an aspect of their behavior in response to an awareness of being observed. In other words, if you expect to be "cured" by a treatment, then you will be.

therapy in treating mental illness is so important that the subject is discussed in Chapter 8 (Aromatherapy for PTSD and depression).

As an aside, the 13 y.o. daughter of a friend of the author was having trouble sleeping and once a lavender oil diffuser was placed in the bedroom, restorative sleep was re-established. The friend mentioned, however, that although her daughter now slept better, she was waking up with migraines. When they switched to Young Living lavender oil for the diffuser, not only were sleep patterns improved but there were no more migraines. This was a clear example of the importance of using only 100% pure, natural essential oils.

Many essential oils, Table 7.2, are widely believed to be effective anxiolytic (anxiety-reducing) agents and most people readily agree that the aromas of these essential oils have a calming, relaxing and soothing effect on the mind and body.

Bergamot
Chamomile
Frankincense
Geranium
Lavender
Lemon
Pine
Rose
Rosemary
Salvia
Sandalwood
Sweet Orange
Ylang ylang

Table 7.2 Anxiolytic (anxiety-reducing) Essential Oils

It should be mentioned that Young Living, for example, has compounded several essential oil blends designed to achieve relaxation, tranquility, anxiety relief and alleviation of stress. Some of these products are indicated in Table 7.3.

Oil Blend	Action
Aroma Ease	Calming Effect
Aroma Siez	Soothing and relaxing
Endoflex	Calming and balancing
Forgiveness	Supports ability to forgive oneself and letting go of negative feelings
Oola Field	Encourages self-worth and overcoming internal barriers
Present Time	Helps focus on the present and diminish past traumas
Release	Helps release anger, frustration and memory trauma, and open the subconscious mind.
Rutavala	Soothes stressed nerves, and induces sleep
Sara	Helps relaxation to facilitate the release of the effects of trauma and physical or mental abuse
Stress Away	Induces feeling of peace and tranquility, helps relieve stress and nervous tension, restores equilibrium, promotes relaxation, and lowers hypertension
The Gift	Calming effect
Trauma Life	Combats stress, anger, restlessness and insomnia caused by trauma
Tranquil	Reduces stress, restlessness and anxiety, has calming and relaxing effect on mind and body, and promotes sleep
Valor	Empowering effect, promoting feelings of strength, courage, and self-esteem
White Angelica	Feelings of safety and security, guards against negative energy.

Table 7.3 Anxiolytic and Relaxing Essential Oil Blends*

*: Formulated by Young Living, Lehi, Utah.

Most of the pure oils and blends listed in Tables 7.2 and 7.3 can be applied directly to the skin (as in massage therapy) although the packaging should be checked to determine whether the pure essential oil or oil blend should be diluted with a carrier oil to avoid skin irritation. This is an important precaution for users with sensitive skins, people with a history of eczema or dermatitis as well as when any essential oil is to be used on babies or young children. There are, however, specially formulated essential oil blends (e.g. Gentle Baby) that are calming for mothers and babies.

There is a growing medical literature on the application of aromatherapy in relieving many of the symptoms associated with dementia. Clinical studies certainly indicate that dementia patients benefit from aroma therapy as do sufferers from many other afflictions that cause stress, insomnia and anxiety-related effects. The scientific basis for this is that when an aroma is inhaled, it will reach and then bind to olfactory receptors. These receptors initiate subsequent events that trigger action potentials (minute electrical impulses) that are propagated up the olfactory nerve to the limbic system[38] in the brain, particularly the amygdala[39]. Since this is the same part of the brain that controls emotion, there will be a direct stimulation of the emotional center in the brain. Other research studies indicate that aromatherapy with essential oils is related to decreased levels of cortisol[40], reduced inflammation, lowered heart rate, reduced anxiety and alleviates depression. In other words, the effects elicited by aromatherapy are likely the result

---

38 The *limbic system* is complex system of nerves and networks in the brain, involving several areas near the edge of the cortex concerned with instinct and mood. It controls the basic emotions (such as fear, pleasure and anger) and human drives (such as hunger, sex, dominance and care of offspring).

39 The *amygdala* is one of two almond-shaped groups of nuclei located deep within the temporal lobes of the brain and is the integrative center for emotions and motivation. The *amygdala* gives rise to fear when we face things outside our control, notably how we react to certain stimuli or an event that is seen as potentially threatening or dangerous.

40 *Cortisol* is the hormone released by the adrenal gland in response to stress and low blood glucose; its actions include increasing blood sugar, suppressing the immune system and aiding in the metabolization of protein, fat and carbohydrates.

of mood changes as well as physiological ones and, further, the mood-based changes may depend on subjective memories that are tied to particular scents.

It should be mentioned, however, that there have been comments that there is no convincing evidence that aromatherapy can relieve hypertension, depression, anxiety, pain or symptoms of dementia. It has been said that although the scent of lavender may have a calming effect in some people and help with sleep, but it can cause headaches in others. The latter effect was mentioned above and might be the result of using a synthetic or adulterated lavender oil. Nevertheless, although the "nay-sayers" and skeptics will admit that scents can be calming and pleasing to people, they maintain these effects may not be due to any biological or pharmacological impact, but rather a sensory or psychological effect. So, as with many things, the bottom line should be that if aromatherapy works for you, then enjoy it regardless of what mechanism might be operating in relieving symptoms.

Finally, it should be mentioned that aromatherapy products do not need approval by the FDA and different aromatherapists use various combinations of oils, and methods of application in their treatments. The differences in oil combinations and blends, as well as the preferred methods of application are practitioner-dependent. Overall some approaches are more widely accepted than others throughout the aromatherapy community, as discussed below.

AROMATHERAPY and MEMORY

As mentioned at the start of this chapter, the sense of smell is closely associated with memory, probably to a greater degree than for any of the other 4 senses. People with full (unimpaired) olfactory function can think of smells that evoke particular memories and, often spontaneously, a particular smell can act as a "trigger" to recall a long-forgotten event or experience. Further, as is well-recognized by the perfume industry, the sense of smell is highly emotive and perfumers and essential oil blenders work hard to develop fragrances designed to stimulate different emotions and feelings, including but not limited to power, vitality, relaxation and even desire.

The association between the sense of smell and the mind is underscored by studies which showed that personal body odor, produced by the genes comprising the immune system, help subconsciously in the choice of life partners. That this suggestion is intuitively correct is probably related to the fact that individual responses to smells are governed, and perhaps determined, by association. This might explain why different people have completely different perceptions and/or reactions to the same scent. Such reactions contribute to the difficulty of quantifying smells, as mentioned above.

The importance of the association between the sense of smell and the mind, notably memory, was studied a few years back by a team of scientists in Germany. In the study, 74 healthy adults aged between 20-30 years, were asked to review pairs of cards jumbled across a computer screen. Some participants were seated at computers in a room perfumed with rose scent whereas the others were seated at computers in unscented rooms. All participants then spent the night at a sleep lab, with electrodes placed on their scalps to monitor brain activity during sleep. While participants slept deeply (slow-wave sleep) or during light REM (rapid eye movement) sleep, their rooms were briefly perfumed with the rose scent.

The next day, study participants took a computerized "pop" quiz requiring them to identify the card pairs they had seen the previous day. Participants who had smelled the rose scent twice, i.e. during the computer session the previous day and during deep sleep (non-REM or slow-wave sleep), performed best on the quiz. However, it was noted that exposure to the rose scent during light REM sleep did not improve test scores.

Interestingly, in a follow-up study, it was found that exposure to the rose scent only during the daytime did not affect test scores. In other words, these research studies indicate that exposure to a scent while learning and again during deep sleep appears to aid the memorization of what people had learned.

Support for this conjecture regarding a scent-memory connection comes from other studies involving 14 participants asked to sleep in a magnetic resonance imaging (MRI) scanner. The participants apparently had participated in past MRI studies, so that they were familiar with the MRI and were able to fall asleep during the study. They also wore earplugs and headphones to reduce noise. The MRI brain scans showed that one particular area of the brain, the hippocampus[41], became particularly active while participants smelled the rose scent during deep (slow-wave) sleep but, evidently, not during REM sleep. The olfactory system apparently activates prior memories in the hippocampus, making it easier to store new data during slow-wave (deep) sleep.

The study findings suggest that the hippocampus may be a key organ or area of the brain involved in building memories by the mind. These studies indicate that scents may strengthen or enhance memorization of information by the brain. This study also might explain the finding that exposure to the rose scent during light REM sleep did not improve test scores in the previously cited research study.

Unfortunately, neither set of researchers tested any other scents to see if the memory-stimulating effect was specific to the aroma of rose or whether similar effects could be found with other scents. Nevertheless, the overall conclusion that can be drawn is that exposure to certain scents at the right time can strengthen recall and that using a diffuser while studying and sleeping improves memory.

ESSENTIAL OILS and THE LIBIDO

Although aromatherapy is effective in inducing calmness and relaxation (see Tables 7.1, 7.2 and 7.3), a curious effect was shared with the author. A new user and strong proponent of essential oils found that putting Young Living's essential oil blend, Joy, into a diffuser had a marked effect on the libido of her husband. Further, this effect was reinforced when 1-2 drops of Joy were placed on the "bridge area" of his shorts.

The Young Living Product Guide indicates that the aroma of Joy invites a sense of romance, bliss and warmth when diffused while its use as a fragrance invites togetherness. To the delight of the lady in question, these "claims" for Joy have certainly proved to be true.

---

41 The *hippocampus* is the organ in the brain that regulates emotions and is associated mainly with memory, particularly long-term memory.

Other products, such as *Live Your Passion* and *Live with Passion* may have a similar effect although no information is available at this time whether this is the case.

AROMATHERAPY and AROMATHERAPISTS

Training courses, and certification, in aromatherapy are available at several institutions throughout the United States and in many other countries. However, there is no professional standardization and no license is required to practice aromatherapy in the USA. As a result, there is little consistency between practitioners in the treatments used for specific conditions. One result of this lack of standardization is that there tends to be inconsistency in research studies on the effects of aromatherapy. In part, this is because tradition, anecdotal evidence and the prior experience of the practitioner combine to determine his or her selection of essential oils. Consequently, the choice of oils by researchers in clinical trials can often be quite arbitrary when studying the same applications. Also, as noted above, the benefits of aroma-therapy are highly subjective which complicates scientific study of this treatment modality.

This situation is now changing, with specific courses being available for healthcare professionals and caregivers wanting to become aro-matherapists. These courses often satisfy continuing medical education contact hour requirements for healthcare professionals and many also include a research component and provide information on evaluating aromatherapy outcomes. As a result, the landscape of aromatherapy has been changing and improving in recent years.

At least two governing bodies, The National Association for Holistic Aromatherapy and The Alliance of International Aromatherapists, are working to establish national educational standards and to standard-ize aromatherapy certification for aromatherapists. The Canadian Federation of Aromatherapists likewise has established standards for aromatherapy certification in Canada and advocates standards for safety and professional conduct. Similar organizations likely exist in many other countries. It should also be mentioned that whereas aromather-apy in the USA is generally limited to inhalation or topical application, aromatherapists in France and Germany often encourage oral use of essential oils. This approach follows the teachings of Gattefossé, Valnet and later practitioners and is based on the belief that there are internal (systemic) benefits from ingesting essential oils.

Finally, although many research studies on aromatherapy have been conducted with synthetic oils, most aromatherapists believe that synthetic fragrances are inferior to pure essential oils because they lack "natural or vital energy". Such comments probably refer to the naturally occurring minor ingredients in pure, natural essential oils. As previously discussed in this book, such comments by experienced aromatherapists are supported by the fact that synthetic oils do not contain the wide variety of "minor" components present in pure, natural oils. On the other hand, this contention regarding the "natural or vital energy" of natural oils has been challenged by psychologists, physiologists and biochemists working in this field although anecdotal evidence suggests otherwise. However, as discussed in several chapters in this book, synthetic essential oils do not contain the many minor components present in 100% ure, natural essential oils. Not only is it likely that these "missing components" act synergistically with each other *and* the major component of the oil, but it is also possible that their effect on the properties of essential oils may be far greater than might be expected from their relatively small content in the oil. It follows from this conjecture that synthetic essential oils may not possess the same properties as their 100% pure, natural counterparts.

CHAPTER 8

AROMATHERAPY for PTSD and DEPRESSION

D
epressive disorders are debilitating and can wreak havoc on the lives of sufferers and their families and loved ones. These mental illnesses take on many forms and include clinical depression, post-traumatic stress disorder (PTSD), post-partum depression and many other conditions. Notes on mental illnesses such as depression and PTSD are given at the end of this chapter, but these notes are included for informational purposes only and should not be used to diagnose or treat any mental illness.

The prevalence of depression is staggering, with over 15 million Americans being affected by the condition every year. Further, depression is the leading cause of disability in the United States (and probably also in many other developed countries) for people in the age range of 15 to 45 years. Interestingly, the median age for the onset of depression is typically 32 years, and it occurs more often in women than in men. Although depression is a readily treatable mental illness, it is estimated that 80% of sufferers either receive no treatment or do not seek help.

Likewise, the prevalence of PTSD is horrifying, with nearly 7.7 million Americans affected by this condition per annum. Most public attention for PTSD pertains to war veterans. However, it could result from common events such as a major accident, natural disaster or personal assault. It has been estimated that among veterans, the prevalence of PTSD is somewhere in the 14-33% range. Although not everyone who experiences a traumatic event will suffer from PTSD, being aware of symptoms and stressors, and even its possibility, may assist with treatment and prevention.

Mood management therapy using pharmaceuticals (prescription medications) is one of the commonest approaches to treating PTSD in a majority of cases in the United States. Today, information regarding integrative therapies is so much more widespread and research substantiating the effectiveness of aromatherapy in treating depression, anxiety and providing emotional support is strengthening. Every one of these symptoms can be associated with PTSD.

Counselling with a skilled and experienced therapist can be of major benefit to sufferers from depression, PTSD and other forms of mental illness. Further, an array of psychotropic/psychoactive medications that can alleviate symptoms are available by prescription, but many sufferers are reluctant to rely on "chemical crutches". So, what does one do when everything appears to be too much to handle and depression settles upon us or even when we repeatedly feel really "down"?

People have used essential oils for centuries to heal the mind and body and their positive effects on us are astounding. Sufferers with PTSD and many other depressive conditions often find that aromatherapy can help them to manage their symptoms. Anxiety-reducing essential oils were listed in Chapter 7 whereas Table 8.1 indicates essential oils that many therapists recommend for sufferers from depression and PTSD.

Bergamot	Anti-depressant effect, reduces stress and tension.
Chamomile	Soothing aroma
Clary sage	Anxiolytic and anti-depressant effect
Geranium	Natural sedative
Lavender	Soothing effect
Lemon	Calming, mood elevator
Pine	Balances the nervous system
Roman chamomile	Anxiolytic and anti-depressant effect
Rose	Tranquilizing effect
Rosemary	Stimulates the circulatory system, reduces fatigue.
Sandalwood	Anti-depressant effect, reduces stress and tension.
Sweet Orange	Tranquilizing effect, reduces anxiety

**Table 8.1 Aromatherapy essential oils claimed
to benefit depression and PTSD**

Once the safe administration of essential oils is established and the oils which provide the best results are identified for the individual patient, then many sufferers find that aromatherapy offers relief from even the most severe depressive conditions, even PTSD. There is certainly a great deal of scientific evidence, commonly known as the *scientific literature*, reporting numerous research studies and patient reactions on the effects of aromatherapy in treating depression and PTSD. Although the mechanism whereby aromatherapy provides relief for sufferers is unclear, the evidence for benefits to patients is increasing daily. In other words, scientific, controlled studies indicate that aromatherapy has great potential as an effective therapeutic option for the relief of depressive symptoms in a wide variety of subjects. It is also interesting that some studies indicate that aromatherapy massage may have greater beneficial effects than inhalation aromatherapy alone.

What is curious is that the beneficial effects of aromatherapy with regard to anxiety, hyperactivity and other symptoms in humans also appears to occur with pets, as discussed in Chapter 10.

CONCLUSIONS

Although the preceding comments were directly primarily at the United States, it is increasingly evident that depression is one of the greatest health concerns known to man, affecting 350 million people world-wide. Aromatherapy is an increasingly popular CAM intervention used by people suffering from depression. This growing popularity of aromatherapy for alleviating depressive symptoms has stimulated numerous research studies and, as stated above, the overall findings are that this treatment modality is effective. However, regardless of the efficacy of essential oils and aromatherapy in alleviating depressive symptoms, essential oil suppliers are prohibited by law from claiming that their products should be used for this purpose. In fact, the FDA mandates that if a product is intended for a therapeutic use, then it is classed as a drug. Therapeutic uses of a product include treating or preventing disease and/or its use to affect the structure or function of the body. Consequently, claims that a product such as an essential oil and aromatherapy will relax muscles, help one sleep or treat depression or anxiety are, in fact, drug claims which cannot and should not be made without successful clinical trials, rigorous testing and FDA approval.

Notes on Depression and PTSD

The following comments <u>are not to be used for diagnosis of mental illness</u>. However, people experiencing many of the common conditions outlined below should seek medical and/or psychiatric/psychological counseling for treatment or to ease their fears.

SYMPTOMS OF DEPRESSION

Depression is a multi-facet mental illness and many sufferers miss the warning signs because their symptoms do not appear to be typical, whatever "typical" might mean! In other words, depression does not present itself in the same way for all people although sufferers may experience many of the classic signs indicated below.

a. Sleep disturbance is a classic sign of depression with some people sleeping too little when depressed, and others sleeping too much. Insomnia or restless sleep can also occur.

b. Major changes in mood such as anxiety, apathy, general malaise or discontent, guilt, feelings of hopelessness, loss of interest or pleasure in most activities, persistent sadness, and sudden mood swings.

c. Behavioral changes such as heightened or atypical irritability, agitation, excessive crying, and withdrawal from society or social isolation.

d. Cognitive behavior: inability to concentrate, loss of interest, reduced activity, lowered self-esteem, dwelling on or frequent repetition of thoughts.

e. Suicidal thoughts.

f. Diminished appetite or minimal interest in food.

g. Significant weight changes – either loss or gain.

Although most of us may experience many of the above symptoms at various times in our lives, particularly when we have experienced major upheavals, it is when these symptoms persist for days, weeks or even years that professional help and support should be sought.

SYMPTOMS OF PTSD

Post-traumatic stress disorder (PTSD) is a mental health condition that is triggered by a terrifying or very traumatic event. The trigger might be an event experienced by the sufferer or it is something that has been witnessed by someone not directly involved in that incident. PTSD may elicit a number of symptoms, including flashbacks, nightmares, severe anxiety as well as repeated and uncontrollable thoughts about that event.

Many traumatic events such as divorce, rape, vehicular accidents, loss of a loved one, job changing and even moving can cause people to experience difficulty in adjusting and coping for a while, but they do not necessarily have PTSD. In many of such cases, time, good self-care and support from family and friends will usually alleviate the symptoms. On the other hand, if the symptoms worsen or last for months or even years, and interfere with normal behavior and functioning, then PTSD may a cause for concern…and treatment.

PTSD symptoms fall into three main classes:

a. Re-experiencing the event, intrusive memories, sleep disorders, intense anger or anxiety at memories of the event.

b. Solitary behavior, detachment, estrangement, numbed behavior, "shutting down".

c. Hyperarousal, nightmares, irritability, sleep disturbance, anger, aggression, impulsive behavior, panic attacks, excessive or atypical response to stimuli.

Most people associate Post-Traumatic Stress Disorder with the military when they return from war or with police officers who have been involved in shoot-outs. But, as indicated above, sufferers from PTSD may include victims of sexual assault, adults who were abused as children, people involved in serious car accidents as well as those experiencing train and aircraft wrecks. People who have experienced traumatic events such as a house fire, severe flooding or other natural disasters may also suffer from PTSD.

Because of the importance of the subjects briefly discussed here and which affect so many of us, a bibliography of medical literature and further reading is provided below.

BIBLIOGRAPHY OF FURTHER READING

Anon. An orally administered lavandula oil preparation (Silexan) for anxiety disorder and related conditions: an evidence-based review. Int. J Psychiatry Clin. Pract. (2013) 17: Suppl 1:15-22.

Anon. Aromatherapy in the management of psychiatric disorders: clinical and neuropharmacological perspectives. CNS Drugs. (2006) 20(4): 257-80.

Conrad P, Adams C. The effects of clinical aromatherapy for anxiety and depression in the high-risk postpartum woman - a pilot study. Complement Ther. Clin Pract. (2012) 18(3):164-8.

Dyer J, Cleary L McNeill S et al. The use of aromasticks to help with sleep problems: A patient experience survey. Complement. Ther. Clin. Pract. (2016) 22: 51-8.

Faturi CB, Leite JR, Alves PB, et al. Anxiolytic-like effect of sweet orange aroma in Wistar rats. Prog Neuropsychopharmacol Biol Psychiatry (2010) 34(4):605-9.

Forrester LT, Maayan N, Orrell M, et al. Aromatherapy for dementia. Intervention Review, The Cochrane Library Published Online: 25 February 2014

Franco L, Blanck TJ, Dugan K, et al. Both lavender fleur oil and unscented oil aromatherapy reduce preoperative anxiety in breast surgery patients: a randomized trial. J Clin. Anesth. (2016) 33: 243-9.

Fung JKKM, Tsang HWH and Chung RCK. A systematic review of the use of aromatherapy in treatment of behavioral problems in dementia (2012) 12: 372–382

Goes TC, Antunes FD, Alves PB, Teixeira-Silva F. Effect of sweet orange aroma on experimental anxiety in humans. J Altern. Complement. Med. (2012) 18(8): 798-804.

Greenberg MJ, Slyer JT. Effectiveness of Silexan oral lavender essential oil compared to inhaled lavender essential oil aromatherapy on sleep in adults: a systematic review protocol. JBI Database System Rev Implement Rep (2017)15(4): 961-970.

Harmon K. Aromatherapy can help PTSD alternative medicinal treatments. Military Spouse (2009) February, pp. 48-49.

Karadag E, Samancioglu S, Ozden D, Bakir E. Effects of aromatherapy on sleep quality and anxiety of patients. Nurs. Crit. Care (2017) 22(2): 105-112.

Kasper S, Müller WE, Volz HP, et al. Silexan in anxiety disorders: Clinical data and pharmacological background. World J Biol. Psychiatry (2017) 19: 1-9.

Kasper S, Volz HP, Dienel A, Schläfke S. Efficacy of Silexan in mixed anxiety-depression--A randomized, placebo-controlled trial. Eur. Neuropsychopharmacol. (2016) 26(2): 331-340.

Keshavarz Afshar M, Behboodi Moghadam Z, et al. Lavender fragrance essential oil and the quality of sleep in postpartum women. Iran Red Crescent Med J. (2015) 17(4): e25880.

Kim W, Hur MH. Inhalation effects of aroma essential oil on quality of sleep for shift nurses after night work. J Korean Acad. Nurs. (2016) 46(6): 769-779.

Lee YL, Wu Y, Tsang HW, Leung AY, Cheung WM. A systematic review on the anxiolytic effects of aromatherapy in people with anxiety symptoms. J Altern. Complement. Med. (2011) 17(2): 101-8.

Maddocks-Jennings W, and Wilkinson J M. Aromatherapy practice in nursing: literature review. Journal of Advanced Nursing (2004) 48: 93–103.

Nikfarjam M, Rakhshan R, Ghaderi H. Comparison of effect of lavandula officinalis and venlafaxine in treating depression: A double blind clinical trial. J Clin. Diagn. Res. (2017) 11(7): KC01-KC04.

O'Malley PA. Lavender for Sleep, Rest, and Pain: Evidence for Practice and Research. Clin Nurse Spec. (2017) 31(2): 74-76.

Press-Sandler O, Freud T, Volkov I, et al. Aromatherapy for the treatment of patients with behavioral and psychological symptoms of dementia: A descriptive analysis of RCTs. J Altern. Complement. Med. (2016) 22(6): 422-8.

Sánchez-Vidaña DI, Ngai SP, He W, et al. The Effectiveness of Aromatherapy for Depressive Symptoms: A Systematic Review. Evid Based Complement Alternat Med. (2017) 5869315. Epub 2017 Jan 4.

Setzer WN . Essential oils and anxiolytic aromatherapy. Nat Prod Commun. (2009) 4(9):1305-16.

Wotman M, Levinger J, Leung L, et al. The efficacy of lavender aromatherapy in reducing preoperative anxiety in ambulatory surgery patients undergoing procedures in general otolaryngology. Laryngoscope Investig. Otolaryngol. (2017) 2(6): 437-441.

Yim VW, Ng AK, Tsang HW, et al. A review on the effects of aromatherapy for patients with depressive symptoms. J Altern. Complement. Med. (2009) 15: 187-95.

CHAPTER 9

MASSAGE THERAPY

Massage therapy is a venerable treatment for relieving muscle and joint pain. In fact, most people will rub aching muscles and joints almost without thinking. Massage therapy is a more formalized approach to relieving aches and pains that is performed by trained and highly skilled professionals. The practice dates back over thousands of years and references to massage have been noted in ancient writings from China, Egypt, India and Japan. It is an important component of Complementary or Alternative Medicine (CAM) health care approaches (see Table 5.2) for the treatment of a variety of pathologies.

According to records compiled by the Centers for Disease Control (CDC), in 2012 about 1.6% of adults with a musculoskeletal pain disorder used one or more CAM modality for treatment.[42] A somewhat higher prevalence of CAM use (50.6%) was seen among persons who had neck problems such as pain or other musculoskeletal complications (46.2%). The popularity and relatively high use of CAM therapies is possibly because in any given year, ¼ to ⅓rd. of adults might be suffering from one or more musculoskeletal disorders. Further, many forms of chronic pain do not respond that well to conventional medical treatment other than analgesics (pain killers). Interestingly, approx-

---

42   National Health Statistics Reports Number 98; Centers for Disease Control, October 12, 2016

imately 1% of adult CAM patients used it to treat sinusitis (1.2%), elevated cholesterol (1.1%), asthma (1.1%), hypertension (1.0%), and/or menopause pain and discomfort (0.8%). Included in the category of CAM therapies (see Table 5.2) is massage therapy and it is estimated that about 18 million U.S. adults and 700,000 children receive massage therapy each year. These numbers apparently are growing year by year.

It should be noted that many cultures have developed their own, almost unique, therapeutic massage techniques. Thailand, China, Japan, India, many Middle Eastern countries as well as Indonesia have all created their own, quite individualized approaches to massage therapy. In general, as discussed below, the Swedish massage technique appears to be the method mostly widely used in the Western world.

MASSAGE THERAPEUTIC METHODS

People seek massage therapy for a variety of health-related issues. As noted above, these include, but are not limited to, pain relief, stress reduction and relaxation, rehabilitation of sports injuries and as a means of relieving anxiety and depression. In general, massage therapists work on muscles and other soft tissues using long strokes as well as kneading, applying deep circular pressure movements and vibration, and often tapping. This massage technique is commonly known as Swedish massage. Sports massage utilizes Swedish massage combined with the application of deep tissue pressure to release chronic muscle tension, a technique primarily used for athletes. Other techniques include deep tissue massage and trigger point massage which focusses on myofascial trigger points. The latter are the so-called muscle "knots" that are painful when pressed and can cause both localized pain and discomfort as well as symptoms elsewhere in the body. The approaches used for stress and pain relief may differ in both style and intensity with the therapeutic massage techniques developed in other cultures.

In massage therapy, the physical work on soft tissues is often performed in conjunction with the application of essential oils so that patients also receive the additional benefit of aromatherapy. This combination of aromatherapy and massage therapy is often referred to as *aromatherapy massage*. The most commonly used essential oils for massage are listed in Table 9.1 although some suppliers of essential oils do compound "massage oils" and Young Living, for example, formulates and markets six different massage oils, including one for sensitive skins. These blends are designed for different and quite specific massage therapy procedures.

Massage therapists who perform aromatherapy massage often have their own favorite essential oil combinations that they use to achieve certain desired effects. When using pure essential oils, they are customarily, but not always, admixed with a carrier oil to promote oil penetration into the skin and reduce any potential skin irritation issues. The primary carrier oils for most massage oils are coconut, castor and argan oils.

Table 9.1 Essential oils commonly used in massage therapy

Basil	Mountain savory
Coriander	Oregano
German chamomile	Palo Santo
Ginger	Thyme
Lemongrass	Valerian
Marjoram	Wintergreen

TRAINING IN MASSAGE THERAPY

Many health care providers receive training in massage therapy and aromatherapy massage, notably physical therapists, osteopaths and chiropractors in the course of their education. In addition, there are about 1,500 or more massage training programs and massage therapy schools in the United States. Most of these training programs are approved by a state licensing board and/or by independent agencies such as the Commission on Massage Therapy Accreditation (COMTA). Licensed/certified massage therapists usually have received at least 500 hours of training, were required to pass National examinations and satisfy specific continuing education (CE) requirements on an annual or bi-annual basis. As a result, when performed by a properly trained therapist and if appropriate precautions are followed, massage therapy should have few serious risks or adverse side-effects. However, even with the most skilled practitioner, there can be temporary side-effects like pain, discomfort, bruising or swelling. Again, although uncommon, aromatherapy massage can be associated with skin sensitivity or even allergic reactions to the massage oils being used.

BENEFITS OF MASSAGE THERAPY

Over at least the past 30 years, there have been many scientific studies that have attempted to evaluate, and quantify, the beneficial effects of massage therapy. Because the perceived benefits of massage therapy are individualistic and highly subjective, it is almost impossible to perform scientific studies that will provide verifiable and reproducible data or research findings that can be evaluated using statistical analysis, the "yardstick" of science. As a result, opinions and data on massage therapy and aromatherapy massage are predominantly consensus-based rather than scientifically validated research findings. Nevertheless, the bulk of evidence indicates that both massage therapy and aromatherapy massage are beneficial in addressing and alleviating pain and other symptoms associated with many different conditions, Table 9.2. Pain management is discussed again in Chapter 12.

Table 9.2 Conditions benefitting from massage therapy/aromatherapy massage

Muscle and joint pain	Fibromyalgia
Back pain	Infant and child care
Osteoarthritis	Asthma
Mental health/relaxation	HIV/AIDS
Anxiety relief	Pain and nausea associated with
Headaches	chemotherapy

Obviously, there are many other applications of this venerable CAM technique, and, despite the absence of valid evidence-based data from scientific research, the overall testimony suggests that there are many health benefits to massage therapy. However, most of these beneficial outcomes have short-term effectiveness and repeat treatment is usually necessary, and on a regular basis, to maintain full and effective benefits. Further, many reports on massage therapy are conflicting. For example, there appears to be little effectiveness with massage therapy for asthma sufferers despite various claims of its benefits in alleviating or preventing asthma attacks.

Likewise, a critical search of the literature for clinical trials involving massage therapy and aromatherapy massage for symptom relief in people with cancer indicated that many studies were of very low quality and questionable validity. Some studies suggested that massage may help relieve short-term pain and anxiety in cancer patients, other reports indicated that aromatherapy massage may provide medium- or long-term relief for these symptoms. Clearly, more research, preferably involving carefully controlled clinical trials, is necessary in this area.

Despite the widespread and increasingly popular use of massage therapy and aromatherapy massage for treating conditions as varied as childhood autism, asthma, HIV/AIDS and cancer pain alleviation, just how these CAM therapies work is unknown. One theory is that the stimulation provided by massage helps block or interfere with pain signals sent to the brain. This is known by various names but commonly as the *gate control theory*. The basis of this theory is that there is a limited amount of sensory input to the brain and anything that constricts or blocks neural pathways will provide pain relief.

Other people have suggested that massage and aromatherapy massage stimulate the release of chemicals known as neurotransmitters in the body, notably endorphins and serotonin. Endorphins are morphine-like chemicals produced by the body which help reduce pain sensations while triggering positive feelings. In simple terms, endorphins often are called the "feel-good" chemicals in the brain and are the body's natural painkillers. Serotonin is a natural mood stabilizer and is involved in many body processes, including wound healing, sleep, eating and digestion as well as helping diminish depression and regulating anxiety. Based on the activities of these neurotransmitters in the brain and throughout the body, their release through massage therapy and aromatherapy massage should be effective in relieving pain and many other conditions such as anxiety and depression.

Regardless of the multitude of anecdotal reports of the benefits of massage therapy and aromatherapy massage, and their widespread and increasing popularity, prospective users should always exercise a degree of caution. First and foremost, when a patient has a medical condition that might benefit from any CAM technique, a qualified health care provider should always be consulted before embarking on treatment and even be consulted on finding suitable therapists. This is particularly true for pregnant women. Likewise, vigorous massage should be avoided by people with bleeding disorders or low blood platelet counts as well as by patients taking blood-thinners, e.g. aspirin, warfarin and apixaban (Eliquis). Likewise, vigorous massage should be avoided at recent surgical sites.

Further, although it should be obvious, massage must not be performed on patients with blood clots, open or healing wounds (including sutured skin), skin infections or weak bones (osteoporotic patients). As indicated above, massage therapy and aromatherapy massage may be beneficial with some cancer patients and those undergoing chemotherapy and/or radiation treatment. However, patients should always discuss any proposed CAM technique or treatment with his/her oncologist before receiving treatment. Certainly, application of pressure directly over tumors is unlikely to be recommended or approved.

Finally, experienced massage therapists often recommend a variety of essential oils and therapeutic massage to alleviate the discomfort and pain associated with the many different conditions shown in Table 9.2. The following table indicates which essential oils are most commonly used for a variety of conditions. These treatments are not FDA-approved, and this information is for informational purposes only.

Table 9.3 Essential Oils used to treat conditions through Massage Therapy

Condition/complaint	Massage therapy oil*
Anti-cancer	Lemongrass, Thyme.
Anti-inflammatory Properties	Frankincense, Myrrh
Antioxidant Properties	Lavender

Brain and Nerve Stimulation	Coconut
Circulation	Black Pepper, Geranium Ginger, Lemongrass, Peppermint, Rose, Rosemary
Headaches	Lavender, Marjoram, Peppermint, Roman Chamomile
Hormone Regulation	Coconut, Thyme
Nausea	Peppermint, Spearmint
Nervous tension	Frankincense, Helichrysum, Lavender, Neroli, Rose.
Pain	Black Pepper, Clary Sage, Ginger, Helichrysum, Lavender, Lemongrass, Marjoram, Peppermint, Petitgrain, Roman and German Chamomile
Sleep	Jasmine, Lavender, Marjoram, Neroli, Roman Chamomile
Stress relaxation	Bergamot, Clary Sage, Frankincense, Geranium, Grapefruit, Jasmine, Lavender, Marjoram, Neroli, Orange, Petitgrain, Rose, Sandalwood, Tangerine, Ylang Ylang.

*: Essential oils are listed alphabetically

CHAPTER 10

ESSENTIAL OILS and AROMATHERAPY for PETS

Although many people consider their pets to be part of the family and often ascribe human-like characteristics to them, what is known as *anthropomorphism*, animals and humans are very different and not just because they have four legs and we have two. Animals react differently from us to essential oils and aromatherapy and what is safe for use around humans is not necessarily the case for our pets.

It must be stressed that pure and undiluted essential oils are very concentrated so that for pets, very small amounts can have major biological effects on every system of their bodies. When animals absorb essential oils by inhalation, ingestion or through skin contact, the oils can rapidly enter the body and blood stream, and then be distributed to various tissues. Cats and dogs lick themselves several times a day for cleaning and grooming and will ingest whatever you have applied to the skin or fur. Consequently, topical application of essential oils can be problematic, and cats are highly sensitive to certain oils, notably cinnamon, oregano, clove, wintergreen, thyme and birch.

Veterinarians <u>should always be consulted</u> before undertaking any form of essential oil therapy. This is particularly true when dealing with older pets. Also, if the animal is on any medication, veterinary advice should be sought before aromatherapy and, particularly, when topical application of essential oils is contemplated. Also, regardless of whether an essential oil has been used on a pet, whenever a person has handled any essential oil, the hands must be carefully washed to avoid transfer to the animal's fur or to anywhere near its eyes or other soft, sensitive tissues.

The bottom line is that 100% pure and undiluted essential oils should not be used on pets, especially on cuts, wounds or broken skin. Essential oils should never be given orally to dogs or cats because some common oils, including eucalyptus and tea tree oil (melaleuca), can cause kidney and liver damage while large doses of some essential oils can result in seizures. Further, essential oils should never be inserted into the ear canal of a feline as they can damage the delicate ear drums and aural nerves of a cat.

The best rule is that despite the many reports in advice columns and blogs that essential oils can treat minor ailments such as itching, rashes, skin and ear infections, fleas and ticks, veterinary advice should be sought before starting treatment. In general, essential oils appear to be safer for large dogs and horses whereas many "experts" maintain that hydrosols[43] are safer for cats, puppies and smaller animals. However, it should be said that hydrosols may be subject to growth of microbes and, therefore, their use on animals and humans may not be prudent.

If topical application is to be used, regardless of the animal being treated, it is advisable always to dilute essential oils with a good quality base oil such as jojoba oil, vegetable oil complex or sweet almond oil. A safe approach is to add 8-10 drops of essential oil to 20 ml of carrier oil.

The quality of the essential oil is important for both humans and pets. A major problem with lower cost essential oils is that they may contain diluents, contaminants or adulterants that can cause serious issues with pets. Lower cost essential oils may be synthetic, and not contain the highly important minor components mentioned in previous chapters. For this reason, only the highest quality 100% pure and natural essential oils should be used regardless of whether we are discussing pets or humans. Not only that, as discussed in previous

---

43 *Hydrosols* are the liquids left over after distilling out the essential oils from plants. As a result, they are more economical than essential oils but still possess healing properties because they contain the essence of the plants.

chapters, it has been stressed that pure, natural essential oils contain a host of biologically active and powerful compounds which interact together. Used correctly, essential oils can become an indispensable part of integrative veterinary medical care.

It is also worth noting that whereas many "natural" pet care products contain the same essential oils as those used for human aromatherapy and aromatherapy massage, these ingredients in pet products are greatly diluted and are considered safe when used as directed. Internal use of essential oils is <u>never</u> recommended for animals. Also, there have been reports that some essential oils, such as basil, clary sage, sage, marjoram, ylang ylang, cinnamon, thyme and fennel, can cause miscarriages with pregnant animals.

The good thing is that several essential oils can provide emotional support and have a calming and relaxing effect on your pets, particularly when administered through aromatherapy.

AROMAS AND PETS

In the same way that veterinary medicine is an unique specialty in medical science, animal aromatherapy should be considered its own field. Regardless of an individual's knowledge and experience in aromatherapy and using essential oils for humans, special care and knowledge is necessary when dealing with animals.

It is interesting that although millions of people in the U.S. are pet owners, there are few validated scientific studies that have investigated the use of aromatherapy for pets. Consequently, it is not clear whether essential oils and aromatherapy have the same effects on pets as for humans. Nevertheless, there is growing evidence that essential oil aromatherapy has many possible desirable effects with pets. These benefits include reducing anxiety and inflammation as well as fighting infections by inhibiting the proliferation of bacteria, fungi and viruses.

The olfactory systems of dogs and cats far exceed those of humans in terms of sensitivity and capability. In fact, the percentage differences in acuity and sensitivity for humans and animals run into the hundreds if not thousands. Cats and dogs use their very sensitive and highly efficient olfactory systems to acquire and evaluate a great deal of complex information about their environment. This gathered information is used to determine responses and behavior in most situations. This is somewhat akin to how people will often smell food to check freshness but what we can do in this regard is far inferior to what our four-legged friends can do with their innate skills. So, the aromas that might be pleasurable, effective and safe for people may be overwhelming for animals.

Consider, for example, how most of us have been upset when exposed to over-use of perfumes and colognes.... how many times have we been almost nauseated by being in an elevator with an overly perfumed individual? This sort of reaction may occur with dogs, cats and even birds when exposed to aromas that adversely affect them. It follows that caution in the use of aromatherapy and essential oils is mandatory around pets. In fact, an "escape route" should always be provided for the first few times that a pet is to be exposed to aromatherapy. This will allow it to leave the room if any given aromatherapy oil causes it distress.

Nevertheless, there is growing evidence that aromatherapy can be very useful and beneficial for our pets.

AROMATHERAPY AND PETS

As with humans, aromatherapy can be used to affect the mental state and behavior of animals. Lavender oil, for example, has a powerful and calming effect on the brain. In fact, small amounts of lavender oil can be used when traveling to calm pets or make them feel sleepy, provided that it is known that the animal can tolerate that aroma. The best way to achieve this relaxation is to put a few drops of the essential oil on a cloth or cotton ball and tape it to the exterior of the carrier. My wife and I have found that our own cats are far calmer and get along much better together when exposed to lavender oil aromatherapy by aerial diffusion. Even the renowned canine expert Cesar Milan has used aromatherapy to reduce anxiety and hyperactive responses in dog patients. It is always worth asking your pet's veterinarian if they have any experience with essential oils and aromatherapy. Some use them on a regular basis and their advice can be very helpful.

Table 10.1 Essential Oils Considered to be Safe for Pets

Essential Oil	Effect/Action
Cardamom	Diuretic, anti-bacterial, normalizes appetite, controls coughs, reduces heartburn and nausea.
Fennel	Supports the adrenal cortex, helps break up toxins and fluid in tissues. Balances pituitary, thyroid and pineal glands.
Frankincense	Supports the immune system and promotes blood supply to the brain (although it can worsen hypertension). Reported to help with some cancers by shrinking tumors and skin ulceration.
German chamomile	Effective against allergic reactions, stings and burns.
Helichrysum	Supports cardiac health, repairs damaged nerves, skin regenerator, reduces bleeding in accidents, anti-bacterial action.
Lavender	Calming effect and also may help with car and motion sickness. Reported to help with allergies, burns, ulcers and insomnia.
Spearmint	Balances metabolism and assists weight reduction; good for colic, diarrhea and nausea.

There are physical and emotional benefits for pets from aromatherapy although the primary use is to calm and relax them. Other benefits include:

- Bolstering the immune system
- Effectiveness in repelling fleas and ticks
- Relieving the discomfort of itchy skins and rashes.
- Helping with joint conditions, digestive problems, respiratory conditions and circulatory issues
- Alleviating emotional issues such as anxiety, nervousness and stress
- Neutralizing the bad odors that can occur with pets.

Ironically, before exposing a pet to aromatherapy with an essential oil, it might be advisable to check that it actually likes the aroma. Before using any essential oil, apply a few drops to a cloth or cotton ball and let the animal sniff the oils and check the reaction. If the animal turns its head away and walks off, then it probably doesn't like what it is smelling. Sneezing, whining, pacing and teary eyes can all be signs that your pet dislikes or is overwhelmed by the aroma. On the other hand, if the pet sniffs the treated material and seems interested, then your pet probably likes or at least tolerates that particular essential oil.

Finally, it should be mentioned again that after a pet owner handles any essential oil, the hands must be carefully washed to remove any traces on the skin. This will avoid any accidental transfer of the oil onto the pet's fur and prevent the animal from ingesting it when licking itself or another animal that has been exposed to the oil. Not only that, it is critical that the essential oils never go anywhere near the eyes, nose, ear interior, anus or any other soft tissues of pets. Animals, unlike humans, cannot rinse away any foreign material that gets on their bodies or into their eyes, etc. Careless use of essential oils on or around pets can cause needless pain and discomfort for our four-legged friends.

CHAPTER 11

OUTSIDE THE BOX

C lassical literature and archeological records clearly indicate the antiquity of essential oils. The ancient Assyrians, Greeks, Egyptians, Romans and many other older civilizations used essential oils in medicine, for perfumes and cosmetics, as well as for aromatherapy and massage therapy. The distillation of rosewater and other components of perfumes, for example, apparently stemmed from Islamic discoveries in the 9th Century AD. These topics have been discussed in many books[21,44,45,46,47,48,49] as well as in several chapters of this book.

---

[21] von Fraunhofer, J. A. *Essential Oils. A Concise Guide*. CreateSpace, Seattle, WA (2017).

[44] James P, Thorpe N.: *Ancient Inventions*. Ballantine Books, New York, NY (2015).

[45] Majno G.: *The Healing Hand,' Man and wound in the Ancient World;* Harvard University Press, Cambridge, MA (1975).

[46] Tisserand, R. *Aromatherapy: To Heal and Tend the Body*. Lotus Press, Silver Lake, WI (1988).

[47] Valnet, J. *The Practice of Aromatherapy*. Healing Arts Press, Randolph, VT (1990).

[48] Wildwood, C. *The Encyclopedia of Aromatherapy*. Healing Arts Press, Rochester, VT (1996).

[49] Keniston-Pond, K. *The Ultimate Guide to Essential Oils*. Adams Media, New York (2017).

The scientific literature contains a multitude of *in vitro* (laboratory) studies that have confirmed ancient beliefs and the precepts of CAM medical practices that the many terpenes, terpenoids and other compounds in essential oils have significant antimicrobial and anticancer activities. However, not all uses of essential oils are directly related to their medicinal effectiveness. In fact, there are many "out of the box" applications that may come as a surprise.

AIR FRESHENERS

Essential oils, almost by definition, are aromatic and this accounts for their continued use in perfumes and cosmetics over the millennia. The importance of essential oils in fragrances has been known since almost the very start of what we know as civilization. Wall paintings as old as 1500 B.C., for example, show that women in Ancient Egypt would place cones of unguents (perfumed fats) on their heads so that over the course of an evening, the fat would melt to deposit a coating of highly scented grease over the wig, clothes and body of the wearer. This practice must have been messy but was probably an effective perfume delivery method.

It is only a small step to appreciate that the pleasant aromas of essential oils could be used to mask the unpleasant odors in houses from so many different causes. These odiferous agents would include human and animal excreta, body odors and the ever-present smells of rotting foods, garbage and waste. Back in ancient times and now in the 21st Century, aversion to bad smells has resulted in the development of odor-masking agents...what we refer to as air fresheners.

The very effective modern air fresheners fall into three main categories: fragrances, odor neutralizers and odor trappers. These odor-eliminating agents accomplish their effects in three different ways:

1. Air fresheners are based on aromatic compounds that mask bad smells, and rely on terpenes, the principal components of essential oils, to achieve their effects. These terpenes include limonene (the primary chemical constituent of several citrus essential oils) and α-pinene (present in pine, juniper and tea tree essential oils). However, it must be stated that opinions

have been advanced that these compounds possibly can react with atmospheric ozone to form carcinogenic formaldehyde.

2. Odor-neutralizing air fresheners contain organic acids, notably maleic and citric acids, which apparently can react with "smelly compounds" to break them down and produce less odiferous molecules.

3. Odor-trapping air fresheners rely for their action on ring-shaped molecules such as cyclodextrins that are made from cornstarch. Apparently, unpleasant odors can get trapped within the ring cavities of these large molecules which prevents them from reaching the nose.

Regardless of the mode of action, most air fresheners are scented (yet another use of essential oils!) but deciding which of these products is the most effective and longest lasting tends to be a matter of conjecture and personal preference.

TOOTHPASTE

Another application of essential oils that takes advantage of their anti-bacterial properties is toothpaste, the scientific term for which is *dentifrice*. Toothpastes are commonly supplied in the form of a paste, gel or powder and all are designed to perform 3 functions when applied with a toothbrush:

1. An abrasive/detergent action to remove debris, plaque and stains
2. A polishing action to increase light reflectance and improve esthetics
3. Facilitate delivery of various therapeutic agents.

The abrasives and detergents in toothpaste polish the tooth surface to improve esthetics *and* promote resistance to the accumulation of micro-organisms and stains. Toothpastes do not need to be highly abrasive to effectively clean teeth since toothbrushes, especially modern electric toothbrushes, are now very efficient in removing plaque and stains. Toothpastes that are accorded the seal of the ADA (American

Dental Association) Acceptance Program must meet specific requirements. These include abrasivity characteristics, scientific data from clinical trials, and packaging claims that indicate what the product does (and does not do).

Plaque is a coating that attaches to teeth and its removal is essential for oral health. This is because plaque contains bacteria (commonly *Strep. mutans*) that cause cavities (dental caries) and gum disease. Unless it is removed by proper brushing and flossing, plaque can harden into calculus (or tartar) on the tooth surface and below the gum line. As both plaque and calculus build up over time, they will cause gingivitis (gum inflammation) and periodontal (gum) disease. However, it must be said that unless the toothpaste contains tartar-control and plaque-removing agents, it cannot perform the important medicinal function of plaque removal. If the manufacturer claims that a toothpaste removes plaque, the law requires that the product in question is subject to FDA rules, contains plaque-removing agents and must conform to strict regulatory guidelines.

An interesting corollary regarding toothpaste is that products that contain essential oils should facilitate control of plaque (and calculus) because of their antibacterial properties. However, as already stated in several places elsewhere in this book, the essential oil must be a natural (not synthetic) oil for the oft-mentioned major and minor ingredients to work their magic and control the bacteria that cause oral diseases such as gingivitis and periodontal disease. With regard to the latter, clinical observations indicate that dentifrices and mouthwashes containing essential oils, e.g. Young Living's Thieves® products, have a remarkably beneficial effect on the gum tissues. When patients switch to Thieves®-brand toothpastes and mouthwash, dental hygienists and dentists have found that the periodontal probing depths (i.e. the pockets between the teeth and gums and an indication of the progression of periodontal disease) will shrink with continued use. This ensures that there is a reduced risk of gum recession and eventual tooth loss. Further, plaque accumulation is also reduced with this treatment regimen and, interestingly, using Thieves Mouthwash® last thing at night prevented "morning breath". It has also been found that Thieves Lozenges® are effective in alleviating oral malodor and there are indications that they may promote periodontal health.

These observations indicate that the essential oils in Thieves® toothpaste and mouthwash appear to improve overall oral hygiene, alleviate periodontal problems and reduce or shrink the gap between teeth, tooth sockets and gums. Although without controlled clinical trials, no reputable essential oil manufacturer can make the health claim that essential oil-containing dental products "cure" periodontal disease, the evidence suggests that this is indeed what happens when they are used on a regular basis.

Although effective brushing will help remove stains, true tooth whitening is only possible when an oxidant like peroxide is present in toothpaste although peppermint, spearmint, and cinnamon bark essential oils can help with stain removal. These ingredients do give the toothpaste a pleasant taste and freshen the mouth and breath.

Many toothpastes contain fluoride to increase tooth resistance to decay (caries) and some also have desensitizing agents to reduce sensitivity to hot, cold and sweet foods. The fluoride in toothpaste increases the decay-resistance of teeth by a chemical interaction with the enamel. This action is similar to the fluoride treatment that dentists perform on children and adults who are susceptible to dental decay, but it is slower acting than the dentist-applied treatment. Nevertheless, brushing with fluoride toothpaste will improve the caries-resistance of teeth.

Desensitizing toothpastes contain both fluoride and usually a chemical agent such as potassium nitrate or strontium chloride. These agents reduce the flow of ions through the dentin (the inner part of the tooth beneath the surface enamel) and cementum (the lower, root portion of the tooth) through to the dental pulp or "nerve". As resistance to ion flow builds up with regular use, sensitivity to hot, cold and sugary fluids is reduced and eventually will diminish and disappear over time.

A new group of toothpastes, known as remineralization dentifrices, are now available and these both reduce sensitivity and promote remineralization of enamel, the latter strengthening teeth and increasing the resistance to dental decay. Both effects are the result of chemical interactions between tooth and toothpaste and their effects build up over time with regular use.

ESSENTIAL OILS for the HAIR and SCALP.

Over 50% of the male population and a steadily increasing number of females are affected by excessive hair loss and this is a major concern for all affected individuals. This hair loss and/or baldness is known by the medical term *alopecia*. Although alopecia occurs with both men and women, it is more common with males and is known as *androgenetic alopecia*. When hair is lost from some or all areas of the body in spots but most commonly from the scalp, the condition is known as *alopecia areata*.

Alopecia has many causes, including stress, poor nutrition, elevated levels of DHT (dihydrotestosterone), hormonal imbalances (particularly with women) and some medications. Hair loss due to cancer treatment is discussed later. Commonly, alopecia results from scalp tissue problems such as dehydration, poor circulation, inflammation and blocked hair follicles. The psychological effects of hair loss are well-known, and many sufferers invest quite heavily in topical hair-restorer products or hair replacement/transplant surgery in the hope of regaining full heads of hair. Although surgery is usually effective, it can be expensive whereas, by and large, most commercial topical hair restorative products are ineffective at best. Consequently, alopecia sufferers tend to accept the status quo or adopt palliative measures such as toupees, wigs or wearing assorted head coverings and it is not uncommon for balding men to completely shave their heads.

Before addressing treatments for alopecia, it might be useful to briefly discuss hair and hair follicles. The latter are groups of cells that surround hair roots, and which have a three-phase "life cycle". In the first or *anagen* (growth) phase, hair starts to grow due to stimulation of the root which occurs through a process in which follicle cells are converted into hair. In the second or *apoptosis* (cell death) phase, cells in the follicle stop being converted into hair. In the third and final phase, the individual hair strand is ejected, and the follicle goes into a rest or dormancy period. With normal hair growth, this 3-phase process is repeated over and over. Abnormal hair growth or alopecia occurs when there is interference with any phase of the follicle lifecycle and, clearly, the optimal approach to treating hair loss is to address follicular health.

Proponents of essential oils and their many uses have long claimed that certain essential oils can cure or at least ameliorate alopecia by their action on both the hair follicles and the scalp. Those essential oils claimed to stimulate hair growth and reverse hair loss are indicated in Table 11.1. These essential oils are usually used with a carrier such as olive, coconut or jojoba oil. The essential oil mixture should be gently massaged into the scalp and then left in place for 1-2 hours or even overnight before it is removed with a gentle shampoo and warm water.

Most *trichologists* (hair and scalp specialists) dismiss the hair-growth claims of essential oils as anecdotal at best or simply old wives' tales. There is, however, a growing body of scientific literature that indicates essential oils may in fact improve scalp health and stimulate hair growth.

Table 11.1 Essential Oils for the Hair and Scalp

Essential oil	Claimed Action
Cedarwood	Stimulates the hair follicles by increasing circulation to the scalp
Chamomile	Soothes the scalp, shines and softens hair and can lighten hair color
Clary sage	Helps regulate oil production in the scalp to prevent dandruff
Lavender	Soothes the scalp, deepens hair follicle depth, thickens the dermal layer
Lemongrass oil	Strengthens hair follicles, soothes itchy/irritated scalps, reduces dandruff
Peppermint	Stimulates the scalp, treats dandruff and head lice, promotes hair growth
Rosemary	Enhances hair growth, thickens hair by increasing cellular metabolism

A recent research study compared the effects of rosemary oil in jojoba oil with the widely used minoxidil solution in the treatment of alopecia over a 6-month period. Both treatments significantly increased hair count and there was no significant difference between the study groups; there were also no differences in the prevalence of dry hair, greasy hair and dandruff found between the test groups. Although the frequency of scalp itching was significantly higher than that at the start of the study for both test groups, interestingly, scalp itching was more frequent with the minoxidil group compared to that for the rosemary oil group. The findings of this study confirmed a much earlier study on the treatment of alopecia areata (hair loss). In this study, termed *aromatherapy* by the authors, essential oils (thyme, rosemary, lavender and cedarwood) in a mixture of carrier oils (jojoba and grapeseed) were massaged daily into the scalp and compared with the effect of the carrier oils alone over a 7-month period. The results showed "aromatherapy" to be a safe and effective treatment for alopecia areata and significantly more effective than treatment only with the carrier oil mixture.

The effect of peppermint oil on hair growth has also been studied but in mice rather than humans. The study compared the effects on hair growth of topical applications of saline, jojoba oil, 3% minoxidil solution and 3% peppermint oil solution over a 4-week period. It was found that the peppermint oil treatment showed the most prominent hair growth effects, notably a significant increase in dermal thickness, follicle number and follicle depth, and there was no effect on body weight gain and food efficiency for the mice. Whether the findings of this study can be equally applicable to humans may be questionable, but peppermint oil treatment may be less expensive and possibly just as effective as the commercial products based on minoxidil.

Recent research studies[50] by an International research team indicate that sandalwood oil, particularly a patented synthetic sandalwood oil (Sandalore®) developed for the cosmetic industry, shows promise as an approach to ameliorating hair loss. The research team studying the effects on hair growth of the synthetic low-cost alternative to natural sandalwood essential oil postulated the existence of olfactory[51] sensors in the skin, i.e. "smell" sensors additional to those in the nasal passages. These "extra-nasal" receptors are thought to be part of an ancient chemosensory signaling system that evolution developed not so much for "smelling" but more to do with the functioning of human skin

---

50   Chéret, J. et al. Olfactory receptor OR2AT4 regulates human hair growth. Nature Communications (2018) 9.1: 3624.

51   The term olfactory relates to the sense of smell (see Chapter 7).

cell physiology and possibly elsewhere in the body. One of these sub-cutaneous extra-nasal sensors, designated as *OR2AT4*, is of particular interest here.

The research team found that activation of the OR2AT4 receptors in the human skin stimulates both wound healing and hair growth. It is thought that the Sandalore molecule couples to the *OR2AT4* receptor on human hair follicle cells and prolongs the 1st or anagen phase, i.e. the active phase, of the hair cycle. At the same time, this interaction shortens the 2nd or apoptosis phase while increasing the production of IGF-1[52], the hair-growth promoting protein in the outer root sheath. In other words, the hair growth stimulating effect of Sandalore is thought to be multi-factorial, i.e. it stimulates the growth phase and retards the cell-death phase of the overall hair cycle.

At this time, it is not clear whether the reported effects of Sandalore on wound healing and hair growth are peculiar to that particular molecule or would also be found with natural sandalwood oil. The advantage of the synthetic molecule, of course, is that it is much cheaper than the natural product but, at present, comparative studies on effectiveness have yet to be undertaken.

Dandruff[53] is a scalp condition that can be both disfiguring and a source of embarrassment. It is most commonly treated with medicated shampoos but natural remedies for treating dandruff are becoming increasingly popular (see Tables 11.1 and 11.2). For example, it has been found that daily use of an experimental hair tonic containing 5, 10 or 15%. lemongrass oil significantly reduced dandruff at 7 days with an even greater reduction being found at 14-days (Figure 11.1). Interestingly, the findings indicate that a lemongrass oil content of 10% appeared to be the optimal level for effective dandruff treatment, i.e. superior to the higher content tonic.

---

52 Insulin-like growth factors (IGFs) are proteins that are similar to insulin and are components of the complex system that cells use to communicate with their physiological environment.

53 Dandruff is the shedding of dead skin cells from the scalp. A small amount of flaking (about 487,000 cell/cm²) is normal as skin cells die but, with dandruff, unusually large amounts of flaking (about 800,000 cells/cm²) together with redness and irritation can occur chronically or due to certain "triggers". Dandruff can be caused by dry skin, poor scalp cleanliness, yeast-like fungus infections and seborrheic dermatitis (a common skin condition that mainly affects the scalp).

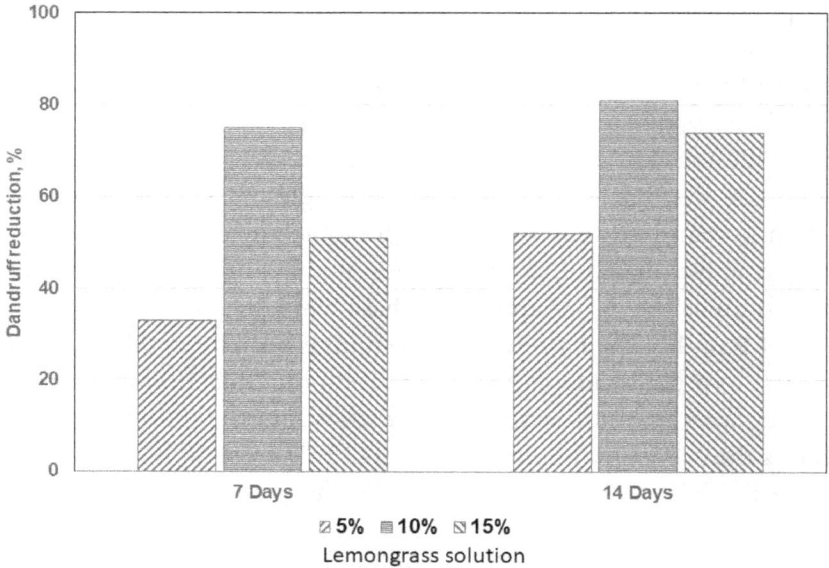

Figure 11.1 Effectiveness of lemongrass oil solution against dandruff.

The studies cited here clearly indicate that essential oils show a great deal of promise for the effective treatment of hair and scalp conditions such as dandruff and alopecia. They also indicate that anecdotal reports of the effectiveness of essential oils in slowing and even reversing hair loss may have a sound scientific basis.

Finally, before leaving this subject, mention should be made of hair loss due to cancer treatment, notably chemotherapy. It is estimated that more than 1.5 million new cases of cancer are diagnosed in the United States each year and these cancers require different forms of treatment, depending upon the type of cancer, its stage and several other patient-specific factors. Approximately 65% of individuals undergoing chemotherapy experience chemotherapy-induced hair loss but this hair loss is usually temporary and completely reversible when therapy ends. The hair loss associated with cancer treatment is related to the selected anticancer agent(s) and the treatment regimen with chemotherapy-induced hair loss most commonly affecting the scalp but sometimes also armpit and pubic hair, eyebrows and eyelashes. Such hair loss can occur within days to weeks of the start of therapy, with complete loss occurring within 3 months after therapy has begun. However, hair often begins to grow back in 1-3 months after cessation of therapy, with some patients finding that the regrown hair may differ in its thickness, color and texture. Generally, hair loss due to chemotherapy is caused by the agent attacking rapidly diving cells in the body, including the dividing hair matrix cells, the latter being amongst the body's fastest growing cell populations. The important thing with this unfortunate side-effect of chemotherapy is that the hair will regrow over time.

FIRST AID

The antibacterial, antifungal and skin-penetrating ability of essential oils has been discussed repeatedly in this book. It is these properties that are the basis for the age-old use of various essential oils for many first aid treatments. Many of these applications are given in Table 11.2 and, for convenient/handy reference, also in Appendix H. Despite the wide-spread and popular use of essential oils and essential oil blends as first aid treatments, the data presented here are for educational purposes only and have not been evaluated by the Federal Food and Drug Administration (FDA). They should not be used to diagnose, treat, cure or prevent any disease.

Table 11.2 First Aid Remedies for Common Complaints

Problem	Conventional Approach	Essential Oils Remedy
Acne	Antibiotics, prescription drugs	Melaleuca*, Lavender
Blisters	Puncture, drain, apply antibiotic cream or petroleum jelly	Lavender
Bruises	Apply ice, elevate	Helichrysum, Geranium, Fennel, PanAway®

Burns	Antibiotic creams, hydro-cortisone, sunlight	Lavender, Geranium, Melaleuca, Myrrh
Colds/sinus/ allergies	Antihistamines, decon-gestants, analgesics	Peppermint, Breathe Again®
Corns	Salicylic acid ointment	Clove
Cuts, skin scrapes, shal-low wounds	Antiseptics, anti-biotic creams	Lavender, Helichrysum, Basil, Melaleuca.
Dandruff	Anti-dandruff, condi-tioner-based shampoo	Rosemary, Wintergreen, Lemongrass.
Depression, anxiety	Antidepressants	Lemon, Frankincense, Peace & Calming®, Stress Away®
Fever	Analgesics	Peppermint
Fungal infections	Prescription antifungal agents, OTC medications	Melaleuca, Cinnamon, Clove, Thyme, Oregano
Headaches/pain	Analgesics	Peppermint, Stress away®
Hives (urticaria)	Antihistamine	Melaleuca, Peppermint
Indigestion, upset stom-ach, nausea	Antacids, Tums®, Pepto-Bismol®	Peppermint, Ginger, Lavender
Inflammation and swelling	OTC anti-inflam-matory medication, Calendula ointment	Frankincense, Melaleuca, Eucalyptus, PanAway®
Insect bites, stings, rashes	Antihistamines, cala-mine, hydrocortisone	Basil, Melaleuca, Melrose, Copaiba, Helichrysum, Roman Chamomile, Purification®

Insect repellant	Chemical sprays, Off®	Citronella, Patchouli, Lavender, Purification®
Insomnia, sleep problems	Unisom®, melatonin, prescription drugs	Lavender, Peace & Calming®
Muscle ache, joint pain	Analgesics, embrocations	Cool Azul®, PanAway®, Deep Relief®
Muscle cramps	Gentle massage, ice and analgesic ointment.	Lemongrass + peppermint, Marjoram, PanAway®
Pain (localized)	Analgesics, Analgesic ointment	Lavender, Eucalyptus, PanAway®, Deep Relief®, Cool Azul®
Parasites	Anti-parasitic and anti-inflammatory drugs	Oregano, Thyme, Fennel, DiGize®
Poison Ivy and Poison Oak	Clean, Calamine lotion, Hydrocortisone ointment/cream	Lavender, Eucalyptus, Cypress, Geranium, Rose, Myrrh, Melaleuca, Joy®
Rashes	Calendula cream,	Geranium, Rose, Lavender
Ringworm	OTC antifungal cream, lotion or powder	Melaleuca, Oregano
Scars	Mederma®, prescription scar creams	Lavender, Frankincense, Helichrysum
Skin cleaning and purifying	Soap, Cetaphil®, Proactiv®, Eucerin®	Basil, Thieves Waterless Hand Purifier®, Thieves Cleansing Soap®, Young Living bath gels.

J. A. von Fraunhofer

Sore throat	Cough drops, throat spray	Thieves lozenges®
Stretch marks	Mederma Stretch Marks Therapy®	Helichrysum, Sage, Rose, Lavender, Neroli, Patchouli
Toothache	Clove oil	Clove, Purification®
Warts	OTC wart ointment	Frankincense, Melaleuca, Oregano, Clove, Thieves®
Wrinkles	Cosmetics	Frankincense

[®: Young Living proprietary oil blend; *: Tea tree oil]

There are, no doubt, many other first-aid (topical) uses of essential oils to treat a wide variety of commonly-occurring skin conditions and irritations. It should also be mentioned that there is increasing evidence that systemic use of certain essential oils can provide rapid relief of several internal complaints and conditions. Whereas such uses appear to be validated scientifically, caution must be exercised whenever essential oils are consumed because they are highly concentrated, and overdosing could cause more harm than good.

CHAPTER 12

PAIN MANAGEMENT

Although the first use of essential oils in pain management is shrouded in antiquity, it is known that Florence Nightingale, the "lady with the lamp" and the founder of modern nursing, used lavender oil on wounded soldiers to control pain during the Crimean War in the 1850s. Since then, practitioners of massage therapy and aromatherapy with EOs have championed the effectiveness of essential oil therapies in pain management. Unfortunately, until comparatively recently, there has been limited scientifically-demonstrable evidence of the effectiveness of essential oils in alleviating pain.

PHYSICAL PAIN

There are two main types of physical pain: neuropathic pain and nociceptive pain, with nociceptive pain being the most common. Neuropathic pain is associated with damage to the body's neurological system, commonly by infection or injury. In contrast to neuropathic pain, nociceptive pain is caused by potentially harmful stimuli being detected by receptor cells (nociceptors[54]) around the body which sense,

---

54 *A nociceptor* is a sensory neuron or nerve cell that responds to potentially damaging stimuli by sending signals via the peripheral and central nervous system (CNS) to the brain. This signaling process, called nociception, induces the perception or sensation of pain.

detect or feel any pain that might be caused by harm to the body. In addition to detecting mechanical or physical trauma or damage to parts of the body such as the skin, muscles, bones and other tissues, nociceptors can also perceive chemical and thermal damage to the body. The former is caused by contact with toxic or hazardous chemicals whereas exposure to extremely hot or cold temperatures leads to thermal damage. Typical causes of nociceptive pain include bruising, burns, sprains, strains, fractures and overuse of muscles or joints as well as exposure to strong acids, alkalis and bleach.

Whereas both types of pain involve transmission of messages to the brain via the central nervous system (CNS), neuropathic pain can manifest in many different ways, possibly because of the abnormal pathways that pain messages follow along the nerves. Neuropathic pain is often described as a "shooting" pain but sometimes may also be described as feeling like a burning sensation along the path of an affected nerve whereas other sufferers may complain of a numb feeling. Further, sufferers may experience neuropathic pain as a constant sensation whereas others indicate that the pain is intermittent, coming and going at irregular intervals. Common examples/causes of neuropathic pain include sciatica, carpal tunnel syndrome, diabetic neuropathy[55] and postherpetic neuralgia (e.g. after subsidence of shingles). Neuropathic pain, known as central pain syndrome, can be caused by multiple sclerosis, Parkinson's disease, brain or spinal cord trauma, or a stroke (cerebral hemorrhage).

Chronic pain is very common, with some 84% of older adults living in nursing homes suffering from persistent, often complex pain. Unfortunately, this chronic pain commonly is not associated with diagnosable conditions although it frequently may be associated with stress and poor coping ability, often leading to other conditions such as poor sleep patterns, anxiety, depression and an overall diminution in QOL.

Pain management by complementary therapeutic means such as aromatherapy, massage therapy and aromatherapy massage were discussed in Chapters 7, 8 and 9. It was mentioned in Chapter 7, for example, that aromatherapy has been shown to decrease levels of cor-

---

55 *Diabetic neuropathy* is nerve damage caused by *diabetes*, typically over time by high blood glucose levels and high levels of fats,

tisol (and possibly increase serotonin[56] levels) in the amygdala and to lower heart rates, reduce inflammation, improve anxiety and alleviate depression. Since anxiety, fear, tension and sleeplessness are linked to pain perception, there is growing awareness of, and public interest in, alternative (non-medicated) approaches to pain management. This desire for natural, effective pain management may in part be a reaction by patients and healthcare providers to the escalating and frightening dependence (and misuse) of opioid-type painkillers.

PAIN and MASSAGE THERAPY

In massage therapy, the physical work on soft tissues is often performed in conjunction with the application of essential oils so that patients also receive the additional benefit of aromatherapy. This combination of treatments often is referred to as aromatherapy massage but for simplicity, the term *massage therapy*, will be used here.

As mentioned in Chapter 9, chronic lower back pain leads to impaired physical activity, lowered QOL and often can lead to reduced productivity and even loss of work for sufferers. The prevalence of both chronic and acute back pain is remarkably high. Some 70–85%, of adults in the U.S. have experienced back pain at least once during their lives, with about 36% experiencing one or more episodes of lower back pain (LBP) each year. Despite non-specific LBP being among the top 5 most common reasons for patients seeking help from healthcare providers, a definitive diagnosis of the cause of pain is possible in less than 15% of sufferers. As a result, getting effective treatment and pain relief can be difficult, and treatment options tend to focus more on the symptoms than the root cause.

Other often severely debilitating and relatively common chronic pains are those affecting the neck and the knee, both of which impact QOL. Causes of neck and knee pain are many and varied, and both commonly are diagnosed as the result of rheumatism and/or arthritis but also due to poor posture, strain or over-exertion. Again, as with

---

56 *Serotonin* is a neurotransmitter, a chemical that transmits messages between nerve cells. It is popularly known as the "happy chemical" because it contributes to overall well-being, mood elevation, appetite, memory, and sleep.

other chronic pains, conventional (non-surgical) treatments for neck and knee pain focus on symptoms rather than the underlying cause(s).

In cases where the cause of severe lower back, knee and neck is clearly established and definitively diagnosed, surgical treatment and, often, prosthetic replacement of severely affected joints can provide sustained pain relief in the worst cases. But, in those cases where a definitive diagnosis is not possible, then sufferers may resort to increasingly potent analgesics and alternative treatment approaches. It should be mentioned here that chiropractic spinal manipulation[57] may often correct problems such as displaced discs or misaligned joints and provide pain relief. However, a single treatment may not always be sufficient to provide extended pain relief and a series of treatments are usually recommended, particularly in cases of trauma-induced misalignments.

Lower back pain: common CAM or alternative treatments for lower back pain (LBP) are chiropractic, acupuncture, routine physical therapy, acupressure and massage, these treatments being directed at correcting the causes. The consensus is that massage, chiropractic and physical therapy are useful for sub-acute and chronic nonspecific LBP treatment, especially if accompanied with exercise. However, massage is more effective than many electrotherapy (e.g. TENS) modalities on their own, and it can be used alone or with electrotherapy for the treatment of patients with low back pain. Other workers have concluded that deep tissue massage (DTM) has a positive effect on reducing pain in patients with chronic low back pain. Concurrent use of DTM and NSAID[58] medications reduced lower back pain to a similar degree to that achieved with DTM alone although another study indicated that DTM provided statistically significant better therapy than conventional massage in pain control.

While there have been many studies of the effect of various massage techniques on LBP, there is little available information on the

---

57 Chiropractic adjustment is performed by medically-trained specialists (chiropractors) using their hands or a small instrument to apply a controlled, sudden force to a spinal joint. This procedure, also known as spinal manipulation, is designed to improve spinal motion and improve spine and neck physical function.

58 *NSAIDs:* nonsteroidal anti-inflammatory drugs are some of the most commonly used pain medicines or analgesics for adults. They are also a common treatment for chronic conditions such as the different forms of arthritis and lupus.

effects on back pain of combining aromatherapy with massage. One clinical trial that compared participants who received Swedish massage using ginger oil with a control group given traditional Thai massage indicated that both groups experienced a significant improvement in pain and mobility. However, pain relief for longer periods of time was reported for the patients receiving massage therapy with ginger oil. Another trial involving acupressure with lavender essential oil over a 3-week course of 8 sessions of treatment for pain relief of subacute and chronic LBP showed a significant reduction in pain intensity and an improvement in lateral spine flexion and duration of walking time ability. It was concluded that acupressure massage with lavender oil may help improve subacute lower back pain.

Although massage therapy shows promise in alleviating chronic low-back pain for patients, some experts in the field have expressed doubt that massage is an effective treatment for LBP. The findings of various studies suggest that whereas massage can effect improvements with acute, sub-acute, and chronic LBP, these improvements in pain control appeared to be only short-term in nature. It should be mentioned also that most scientific articles dealing with LBP indicate that regular exercise is important in dealing with this condition.

Neck pain can be very debilitating and is one of the top five chronic pain conditions in terms of prevalence and work time "lost" to disability. On the other hand, neck pain receives far less research funding than that given to LBP and few clinical trials are dedicated solely to neck pain. Although most acute episodes of neck pain resolve spontaneously, over one third of affected people still have low grade symptoms or recurrences more than one year later, apparently regardless of the treatment received. It appears that nearly half of sufferers with chronic neck pain have mixed neuropathic-nociceptive symptoms or predominantly neuropathic symptoms, with genetics and psychosocial factors being risk factors for persistence of pain. Muscle relaxants and NSAIDs as well as chiropractic and physical therapy can be effective for acute neck pain. Among CAM treatments (see Chapter 5), the evidence is that exercise may provide the greatest relief for chronic pain, with massage, acupuncture, yoga being less effective.

An experimental study compared the results for patients treated with acupoint electrode stimulation combined with aromatherapy acupressure in addition to conventional treatment against those receiving only conventional treatment for neck pain. After 8 lavender oil acupressure and acupoint stimulation sessions, this group reported improved range of motion, lowered pain, reduced stiffness and diminished stress a month after treatment compared to those receiving conventional treatment. These results clearly indicate that aromatherapy is a viable option as a complementary therapy in addition to conventional treatment for neck pain.

Chronic Knee Pain is another common pain experienced by adults aged 50 and older, and it often leads to functional impairment and reduced QOL. As with other types of chronic pain, conventional treatments for knee pain mainly focus on symptoms rather than the underlying cause, and many sufferers resort to CAM for pain relief.

In a double-blind[59], placebo-controlled experimental study of knee pain, massage with ginger oil was compared to the effects of massage only and a conventional knee pain treatment (the control groups). At the 1-week follow-up, knee pain and stiffness were similar among all 3 groups but at 4 weeks, the aromatherapy group reported a reduction in knee pain and an improvement in physical function compared to the control groups. However, none of the participants in the 3 groups reported a significant change in QOL. Despite the study appearing to yield inconclusive results, the researchers suggested that aromatherapy could be useful as an adjunct to standard care in treating knee pain.

PAIN and AROMATHERAPY

Pain management by complementary therapeutic means such as aromatherapy has been discussed in earlier chapters of this book. It was mentioned in Chapter 7, for example, that aromatherapy has been shown to decrease levels of cortisol (and possibly increase serotonin levels) in the amygdala and to lower heart rates, reduce inflammation, relieve anxiety and alleviate depression. Since anxiety, fear, tension and

---

59   A blind or blinded-experiment is one in which information about the test is masked from the participant, to reduce or eliminate bias until all the data is collected and analyzed. If both the tester and subject are "blinded", the study is called a double-blind experiment.

sleeplessness are linked to pain perception, there is growing public and healthcare provider interest in alternative (non-medicated) pain management.

Evidence is mounting that aromatherapy (and aromatherapy massage) with essential oils can be very helpful in managing arthritis pain, labor pains, menstrual discomfort and pain, migraines and chronic pain as well as in treating such symptoms and conditions as anxiety, depression, headaches, respiratory problems and sleep disorders. A recent systematic and meta-analysis[60] of the scientific literature[61] clearly showed that aromatherapy can successfully treat pain when combined with conventional treatments. The study found a significant positive effect for aromatherapy in reducing pain and the authors recommended that aromatherapy should be considered a safe addition to current pain management procedures as no adverse effects were reported in any of the studies they reviewed. Further, the cost associated with aromatherapy is far less than that associated with standard pain management treatments.

Up to 60% of patients who experience hemiplegia (complete paralysis of half the body) after a stroke complain of shoulder pain. Hemiplegic shoulder pain (HSP) is usually caused by muscle weakness, subluxation (incomplete or partial dislocation of a joint) and decreased motor strength. HSP is commonly treated with pharmaceuticals but their side-effects often can be unpleasant and dangerous whereas non-pharmacological treatments, such as exercise, massage and biofeedback can reduce pain but may not always be effective. However, a pilot study back in 2007 looked at the benefits of lavender, rosemary, and peppermint oils on relieving HSP, the experimental treatment group receiving aromatherapy acupressure for 20 minutes twice a day to manage pain. Pain levels in the treatment group were compared to a control group receiving only acupressure without aromatherapy. Although pain was

---

60   Meta-analysis: the term given to the examination of data from a number of independent studies of the same subject to determine overall trends and investigate the consistency of treatment effects across different studies.

61   S. E. Lakhan, H. Sheafer, and D. Tepper. The Effectiveness of Aromatherapy in Reducing Pain: A Systematic Review and Meta-Analysis. Pain Res Treat. (2016) 8158693. Published online 2016 Dec 14.

reduced in both groups, the aromatherapy group experienced a 30% reduction in pain compared with only 15% in the control group, a significant difference in outcome.

PAIN MANAGEMENT in OTHER SITUATIONS

Most people are aware that pain and elevated blood pressure are common after surgery and although analgesics and other medications can reduce pain and nausea, the associated side-effects can prolong the healing process and increase hospitalization time. Aromatherapy is effective in pain management with no untoward side-effects. One study examining pain management after total knee replacement surgery found that patients treated with eucalyptus aromatherapy experienced significantly less pain and lower blood pressures than the control group. Another study that evaluated lavender aromatherapy in patients following breast biopsy surgery found that the aromatherapy group had significantly greater satisfaction with their pain management than the control group, even though the pain levels, use of narcotics and discharge times were the same for both groups.

Pediatric pain management is often difficult because medications like sedatives and opioids commonly prescribed for adults can severely affect brain development in young children. Not only that, pediatric patients in severe pain often refuse to eat or drink fluids which, in turn, can cause dehydration. Another complication with very young patients is their inability to accurately describe the pain they are feeling to caretakers and it is common for children being treated for serious illnesses to experience "distress" not directly related to their illness. These considerations have resulted in a more holistic approach to pediatric care. One study which looked at treating infants with lavender oil aromatherapy for pain caused by taking blood samples showed that infants in the aromatherapy group were soothed faster than those in the control group despite there being no apparent differences in the pain associated with blood drawing. In another study of children recovering from tonsillectomy, those treated with lavender oil aromatherapy slept better and required 40% less of the analgesic acetaminophen than children in the control group. On the other hand, children who had to undergo craniofacial surgery apparently derived no benefit from aromatherapy/

massage therapy. This contrary finding was explained, at least in part, as being due to the children being afraid of strangers massaging them or possibly because massage therapy was applied too soon after general anesthesia.

Complementary therapies, such as aromatherapy, are becoming increasingly common in palliative care and cancer treatment units, with about three-quarters of UK hospitals offering aromatherapy or massage to hospice and cancer patients. Although there are few scientifically valid studies, patient reactions indicate that aromatherapy does reduce pain and alleviate anxiety and depression as well as increasing their overall sense of well-being. These reactions combined with the low cost and easy application make aromatherapy a highly viable option for increasing patient comfort and reducing the use of pain medications for cancer patients.

Although it has been concluded that, overall, aromatherapy provides short-term benefits for anxiety, depression, disturbed sleep patterns, pain and overall well-being, many of the reported studies apparently found no significant differences between aromatherapy and control groups. On the other hand, many studies reported in the scientific/medical literature were poorly designed, had inadequate controls and, often, used essential oils of inconsistent and possibly poor quality. Any, if not all, of these factors would limit the validity and usefulness of the generated data. However, a randomized controlled study involving 17 homecare hospice patients diagnosed with cancer concluded that patients treated with lavender oil reported improved symptoms compared to those with placebo. Further, only members of the lavender group chose to continue treatment after the study. It is not clear, however, if pure essential oils were used in this particular clinical trial. Finally, a different study looked at but did not find any significant long-term benefits of aromatherapy or massage alone in reducing anxiety or pain although statistically significant improvements in sleep scores and reduced depression were reported.

AROMATHERAPY in LABOR

Childbirth and labor are natural processes and, obviously, are essential to the survival of the human race. Nevertheless, the pain of labor can be intense, and may be exacerbated by anxiety, tension and fear. Further, surgical intervention during labor can increase the risk of childbirth complications due to infection, hemorrhage and thrombosis emboli. Because many women are concerned about the effects of pain medication on themselves and their infants during childbirth, natural deliveries are becoming more common. Many mothers-to-be prefer to labor without resorting to drugs or epidural injections and, consequently, turn to complementary therapies to help reduce pain perception. In fact, it is estimated that, worldwide, some 50% of women of reproductive age use complementary therapies for a variety of conditions, including during childbirth. Given the emotional upheavals associated with labor and childbirth, taking advantage of the anxiolytic effects of aromatherapy would appear to be an obvious choice for women. Not only is aromatherapy natural, it is far cheaper and considerably safer than prescription anxiolytic medications and invasive procedures such epidural injections. In addition to managing pain, aromatherapy during labor and delivery may also decrease nausea, vomiting, headaches, hypertension and pyrexia (fever or hyperthermia). As a result, aromatherapy is becoming a frequently requested nonmedical method of managing pain and promoting relaxation during childbirth.

The literature on aromatherapy and labor/childbirth is somewhat conflicted. A review of two clinical trials published in 2012[62], one with 535 women and the other with 22 participants, indicated that no differences were found in pain intensity or the length of labor between the use of aromatherapy, a placebo and no treatment or other non-pharmacological pain management. However, the findings of subsequent clinical studies have challenged and refuted the conclusions drawn in that review as being out-of-date.

---

62 Jones L, Othman M, Dowswell T, et al; Pain management for women in labour: an overview of systematic reviews. Cochrane Database Syst Rev. (2012 Mar)14 (3):CD009234.

One website (Evidence Based Birth: Aromatherapy during Labor for Pain Relief) reported on a large study that followed more than 8,000 mothers at a British hospital in the 1990s. All of the women gave informed consent to the use of aromatherapy during labor and 60% of the participants were first-time mothers with about one in three having their labors induced. In consultation with an aromatherapist, 10 different oils were used in the study. The trial outcomes were compared with the post-delivery comments of roughly 16,000 mothers who did not use aromatherapy on that maternity unit during the same time period. It was found that more than 50% of the women rated the use of aromatherapy as helpful during labor whereas only 13% said that it was unhelpful. It appears that, overall, only 1% of the mothers reported adverse effects from aromatherapy, describing symptoms that included nausea and itchy rash, headache and fast labor. Since these symptoms are consistent with what many mothers normally experience during labor, the authors questioned whether the observed effects were due to the essential oils or if they were just a normal part of labor. There were no reports of any adverse health outcomes for mothers or babies. Further, participants rated rose oil as the most helpful overall whereas peppermint oil was reported as being the most beneficial in dealing with nausea and vomiting.

A clinical study performed in Iran studied the use of aromatherapy with essential oil of orange to control anxiety and stress of women during labor. Although no significant change was found in the physiological parameters (i.e. blood pressure, respiration and pulse rate) of women in the aromatherapy group after the intervention, a statistically significant drop in anxiety was observed.

Other clinical studies, performed in Iran and Thailand, also found that aromatherapy reduced pain and anxiety during labor although apparently it made no difference in the late active phase when the mothers were approaching the end of labor. Although several studies were performed, different modes of treatment were applied and used different essential oils. Most applied the EO by a piece of gauze or a napkin attached to the mother's clothing, adding new drops of essential oil at different points during labor. One study used an incense mask that was held about 20 centimeters (8 inches) away from the participant's face whereas another massaged the oil into the woman's palm. A different study used a warm foot bath containing essential oils for the women in labor whereas yet another diffused essential oil into the air. The essential oils used in the various studies were rose, lavender, citrus, geranium, sweet orange peel, jasmine, *Salvia officinalis*, and bitter orange with the participants deciding which oil they would prefer. All these aromatherapy approaches and essential oils were found to be effective in relieving anxiety and controlling pain, but no comparisons could be made, i.e. no meta-analysis was possible, because of the significant procedural differences in the trials.

The overall conclusion that can be drawn from these different clinical studies is that aromatherapy does reduce pain and anxiety during childbirth. Interestingly, it was noted that aromatherapy with *Salvia officinalis* may help shorten labor whereas geranium essential oil therapy appeared to lower diastolic blood pressure. Because of the significant positive effect of aromatherapy in reducing pain and absence of any adverse effects, various workers suggest that aromatherapy should be considered a safe addition to current pain management procedures during labor. Further, the cost associated with aromatherapy is far less than that for standard pain management treatments and one study found that the cost of providing aromatherapy during labor would only be about $500 to treat 3,000 women!

Finally, in another clinical trial performed in Iran, 140 women admitted to the obstetric and gynecological unit of a hospital were randomly divided into aromatherapy and non-aromatherapy groups immediately after delivery. Intervention with aromatherapy consisted of inhaling three drops of lavender oil every 8 hours for 4 weeks whereas the control group received only routine care after discharge. Stress, anxiety and depression were significantly lower in the study group compared with the control group. In other words, it was concluded that inhaling the scent of lavender for 4 weeks can prevent stress, anxiety and depression after childbirth. This is an important finding since post-partum depression can be quite prevalent, and very debilitating.

POST-CESAREAN SECTION and EPISIOTOMY PAIN

Pain following surgery is a common complaint, and safe and effective pain control after cesarean section (C-section) is important to the physical and mental well-being of both mother and baby. Clinical trials have established that lavender aromatherapy is effective in reducing pain after cesarean section and, in fact, mothers provided with lavender oil aromatherapy had a 90% satisfaction rate with their treatment compared to only 50% in the placebo group. Further, although heart rates were the same in both groups, the lavender group experienced less nausea and dizziness. Because lavender oil aromatherapy effectively reduces pain after cesarean section, its routine use as part of a multi-modal pain management is becoming customary.

Episiotomy[63], a common obstetrical procedure around the world, is used to prevent lacerations and trauma during vaginal childbirth. A sitz bath (soaking in a warm or hot water tub to promote wound healing) is a common treatment recommended by midwives and physicians after episiotomy. At least one clinical trial compared a conventional sitz bath with one containing lavender oil. Although the lavender treatment did not reduce pain, it did reduce inflammation and redness. Another study found that women who used lavender oil for episiotomy pain required fewer analgesics for pain management compared to controls.

MENSTRUAL PAIN

Menstrual pain is extremely common, affecting 25–97% of women worldwide. In fact, menstrual pain for about 15% of adolescents and young women can be so severe that it can stop them from going to work, attending college or school, playing sports or enjoying other activities.

In one study, the menstrual pain of women being treated with abdominal aromatherapy massage was compared with a control group

---

63 *Episiotomy,* also known as perineotomy, is a surgical incision of the perineum and the posterior vaginal wall performed by a midwife or obstetrician; it is usually performed during the second stage of labor to quickly enlarge the opening for the baby to pass through.

of women treated with acetaminophen. Although the aromatherapy group reported a significantly higher rate of relief than the acetaminophen group, it is possible that massage alone might have alleviated the pain. On the other hand, a later controlled randomized blind clinical trial compared an aromatherapy massage group with a placebo group that received massage with no therapeutic oil, and it was found that the aromatherapy group reported a considerable improvement in pain compared to the control. Although there are no data on the effectiveness of aromatherapy without massage on menstrual pain, it is likely to be helpful due to its stress-relaxation effectiveness.

ESSENTIAL OILS in PAIN MANAGEMENT

Overall, the scientific literature does indicate that both aromatherapy and massage therapy are beneficial, i.e. are effective, in pain management. Based on what can be discerned from valid, i.e. controlled, clinical studies, it appears that there are several essential oils, Table 12.1, that effectively manage pain in many different situations. Although many other oils may provide pain relief, those listed in the table have been reported in many clinical trials and anecdotally as being the most effective, with lavender oil situated at the top of the list. It also appears that the onset of pain relief occurs within 30 minutes and that the effects may last for many hours.

Bergamot
Cinnamon
Citrus
Eucalyptus
Geranium
Ginger
Jasmine
Lavendera
Lemongrass
Peppermint
Rose oil
Rosemary
Sweet orange
Salvia officinalis

Table 12.1 Essential Oils providing pain relief in aromatherapy

As discussed in this chapter as well as in earlier chapters, there are various ways in which essential oils may be used in pain control and, clearly, these different approaches incorporate aromatherapy, massage therapy and sometimes a combination of both as in aromatherapy massage:

1) An aerial diffuser (nebulizer) for use in a closed room
2) Pocket inhalers containing essential oils
3) Inhaled aromas by gentle sniffing an open bottle or a cloth on which a few drops of oil have been dripped
4) Using a mister to spray the EO into the air or onto clothing or linens
5) Diluting the EO with a carrier oil and dabbing it onto the skin
6) Adding essential oil to warm-hot bath water (note: bathing in very hot bath water can be injurious)
7) Aromasticks (rattan, bamboo or similar rods placed in a reservoir of essential oil) to act as passive room aerial diffusers
8) Massaging diluted EO into the skin and, particularly, painful joints or muscles

Of course, as already mentioned in previous chapters, undiluted essential oils should not be applied directly to the skin and patch (sensitivity) testing before use is always advisable. Note also that exposure time to certain aromas, as with modalities (2), (3) and (5) above, should be limited to ensure that the olfactory nerves are not overloaded, which might cause the beneficial effects to be diminished or lost. In other words, intermittent use might be advisable.

Finally, many essential oils are recommended by practitioners and blog writers for easing pain and, as previously mentioned, virtually every therapist has his/her preferred individual oils or blends to achieve specific effects. Many of these single oils and blends were cited in Tables 7.1, 7.2 and 7.3, and as indicated in these tables and elsewhere within this book, one or more oils may be recommended for the same symptoms or conditions by different practitioners. Consequently, selection of a given essential oil, and the method of use for any given objective or specific type of pain often comes down to a matter of personal preference for the patient and therapist since not everyone reacts in the same way to the same scent.

CHAPTER 13

SKIN CARE

E ssential oils have been used over thousands of years for medicinal purposes, aromatherapy and cosmetics, as discussed in Chapter 4 and 5. Although, the ancients were aware of the benefits of essential oils in skin creams and cosmetics, most applications were based on trial-and-error observations rather than science. This situation now has changed a great deal.

The skin is the largest organ in the human body and anything that adversely affects the skin is, quite literally, bad for us, a good example being the aggressive and potentially lethal skin cancer, melanoma. The skin, our primary barrier against insults to the body, is bombarded on a daily basis by radiation, pollution and grime, all of which damage our dermal protection. Further, because of air conditioning and "dry heat" from central heating, car heaters and space heaters in offices, stores and workplaces, our skin suffers dryness almost 24 hours a day.

Throughout the 20th Century and now well into the 21st Century, we are inundated by advertisements for skin creams, moisturizers and shampoos, dietary guides and numerous articles on healthy living. These advertisements together with numerous health blogs overwhelm us with adverse comments about free radicals and the damage they can cause to the skin and body. These sources of advice carry lots of information regarding the benefits of antioxidants in counteracting free radicals, with various fruits and vegetables together with numerous dietary supplements being touted as major sources of antioxidants. Although many claims are made for protection against skin cancer, myriad systemic cancers and many other diseases, little information is provided on what free radicals are or how they attack the body.

FREE RADICALS

Free radicals are reactive oxygen and some nitrogen species that are generated within the body and the skin by various internal (*endogenous*[64]) systems, but they also arise through exposure to different physiochemical conditions or various pathological states. The skin is constantly exposed to environmental oxidative stressors such as ultraviolet radiation, air pollutants, chemical oxidants and various microorganisms. In fact, reactive oxygen species (ROS) are considered major contributors to skin aging, cancer and other skin disorders, and they are also a major factor in systemic cancers as well as the aging processes within the body. The mechanism whereby free radicals cause damage to cells of the skin and body is quite complex and beyond the scope of this book, but the bottom line is that they react negatively with DNA, proteins and lipids.

The human body has several enzyme systems that scavenge free radicals, but its principal defense against free radical attacks are antioxidants. The latter are molecules that interact with free radicals and stop their actions before they can damage vital components in the skin and within the body. The body acquires these antioxidants from certain vitamins and minerals, notably vitamin E, beta-carotene and vitamin C as well as the metalloid selenium.[65] These micronutrients are not produced within the body and they must be supplied in the diet. This need for dietary antioxidants is the basis for the often-uttered advice to regularly eat fruit, vegetables and/or consume assorted vitamin and mineral supplements.

Interestingly, the body requires a balance between free radicals and antioxidants to function properly but if the level of free radicals is

---

64   Endogenous systems or agents are internally derived within the body whereas exogenous agents originate or are produced from outside an organism, tissue or cell.

65   J. A. von Fraunhofer. Vitamins, Minerals and Spices. Kindle/CreateSpace, Seattle, WA. (2013).

sufficient to overwhelm the body's ability to regulate them, a condition known as *oxidative stress* can occur. A consequence of oxidative stress is that the "excess" free radicals will attack lipids, proteins and DNA in the skin and body, initiating many diseases, aging and pathologies such as cancer.

When healthy, the skin has an innate antioxidant defense system, but this can be overwhelmed by free radicals, ultra-violet (u.v.) light, and various pollutants and oxidants. Unfortunately, the skin's antioxidant capacity can be depleted when excessive free radical attack occurs and, as a result, important biomolecules such as lipids, proteins and nucleic acids are damaged. With continued exposure to the ROS sources, the onslaught leads to oxidative damage, skin cancer, immunosuppression and premature skin aging. One approach to preventing or at least minimizing ROS-induced photoaging is through the topical application of exogenous antioxidants to the skin to support its natural (endogenous) antioxidant system. Sunscreens will reduce the damage caused by the ultra-violet rays in sunlight, but they can do little against the other environmental sources of ROS. This is where cosmetics come in.

PROTECTING THE SKIN

The antibacterial and antioxidant properties of essential oils were mentioned in Chapters 4 and 5. The topical antibacterial efficacy of essential oils arises from their skin-penetrating ability, and it is this property that accounts for their antioxidant capacity and functionality, notably their role in preventing cellular damage to the skin. Taking advantage of this property of essential oils in cosmetics has been the subject of detailed scientific studies performed in various parts of the world, notably Italy[66,67].

In recent years, amongst the most commonly used ingredients in OTC (Over the Counter) antiaging cosmetic preparations are essential oils. The interest in formulating cosmetics with essential oils is logical

66   P. Ziosi, S. Manfredi, S Vertuani, et al. Evaluating essential oils in cosmetics: antioxidant capacity and functionality. Cosmetics & Toiletries (2010) 125: 32-40.

67   R. Amorati, M. C. Foti and L. Valgimigli. Antioxidant activity of essential oils. J. Agricultural and Food Chemistry (2013) 61: 10835–10847.

in that they are nontoxic and have outstanding antioxidant potential. So, users and formulators of cosmetics and skin creams recognize not only that essential oils will modulate certain types of environmental damage to skin through their antioxidant properties but also that there is a world-wide growth in the appeal of natural and organic products for consumers. Further, there is growing awareness that the most common and widely used synthetic antioxidants incorporated in cosmetics, notably butylated hydroxyanisole (BHA) and butylhydroxytoluene (BHT), are suspected of being potentially harmful to human health. In fact, not only do the FDA and the Environmental Working Group issue warnings about many of the ingredients collectively termed "fragrances" in cosmetics, the European Union and the European Commission on Endocrine Disruption also indicate that certain "fragrances" and ingredients in cosmetics interfere with hormonal function and can even promote the growth of tumors. In other words, natural is better and safer than many synthetic compounds present in cosmetics. This topic will be returned to in Chapter 14, Adverse Effects.

Because natural essential oils are mixtures of numerous components, different types of antioxidants or oxidizable terpenoid components often coexist within a single oil. When a natural essential oil is used as a skin protection ingredient, it is commonly thought that the most effective antioxidant components dominate, and that they provide the greatest protection. Whereas this is true in some cases, there are many exceptions. In fact, the overall antioxidant performance of an essential oil is the result of the complex interplay between the essential oil's components and the skin.

There is now an increasing interest in incorporating pure essential oils in soaps and skin cleaners as well as in after-shave lotions and shaving creams. Young Living, for example, markets several different toiletry products that take advantage of the natural skin softening, moisturizing and purifying action of essential oils. The fact that wholly natural (i.e. non-synthetic) ingredients are used to formulate such products has a major appeal for consumers. The moisturizing, softening and emolient action of certain essential oils, notably helichrysum, age, rose, lavender, neroli and patchouli oils, may also have great appeal to women in dealing with stretch marks after pregnancy and giving birth.

Studies indicate that good antioxidant behavior can be expected from essential oils with a large content of phenolics and a lower content of unsaturated terpenes; even greater protection could come when the oil contains both large amounts of phenolics and a significant content of components like γ-terpinene.[68] Essential oils with little or no content of phenolics and cyclohexadiene-like components such as γ-terpinene are unlikely to provide good antioxidant protection.

It should also be noted that the antioxidant activity of essential oils is based on their principal component and, notably, on their content of minor components. As previously discussed, these may be affected by the botanical source (wild-grown or cultivated plants), environmental and climatic factors. Accordingly, antioxidant activity can vary depending on where the plants were grown, seasonal variations during growth and the way the plants were farmed and harvested. The extraction process may also influence the antioxidant capacity of the essential oil. Finally, it follows that synthetic essential oils, which do not contain the large numbers of minor components found in natural oils, are unlikely to possess the notable and highly important antioxidant capacity found with the pure natural oils.

SOAP, BODY WASH and SHOWER GEL

Soap, body wash and shower gel all contain surfactants or "wetting agents". These are molecules with one end that dissolves in water whereas the other end dissolves in oil and grease. The water-dissolving end has the scientific term hydrophilic (i.e. water-loving) whereas the oil-dissolving end is hydrophobic or water-hating. The term lipophilic or fat-attracting may also be used for the "business end" of the soap/surfactant molecule.

In simple terms, this can be shown in Figure 13.1 as follows:

---

68   *Gamma-terpinene* (γ-terpinene) is a natural hydrocarbon extracted from various plant sources, notably citrus fruits, with a lemon odor and strong antioxidant activity. It is widely used in foods, flavorants, soaps, cosmetics, perfumes as well as in pharmaceuticals and confectionery.

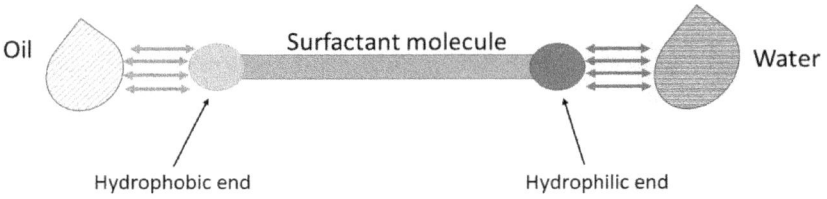

Oil — Surfactant molecule — Water

Hydrophobic end   Hydrophilic end

Figure 13.1 Schematic representation of the action of a surfactant

The hydrophobic ends of the surfactant molecules will become imbedded in to the oil or grease whereas the hydrophilic end is attracted to the water in which the oil/grease globules are suspended, Figure 13.2:

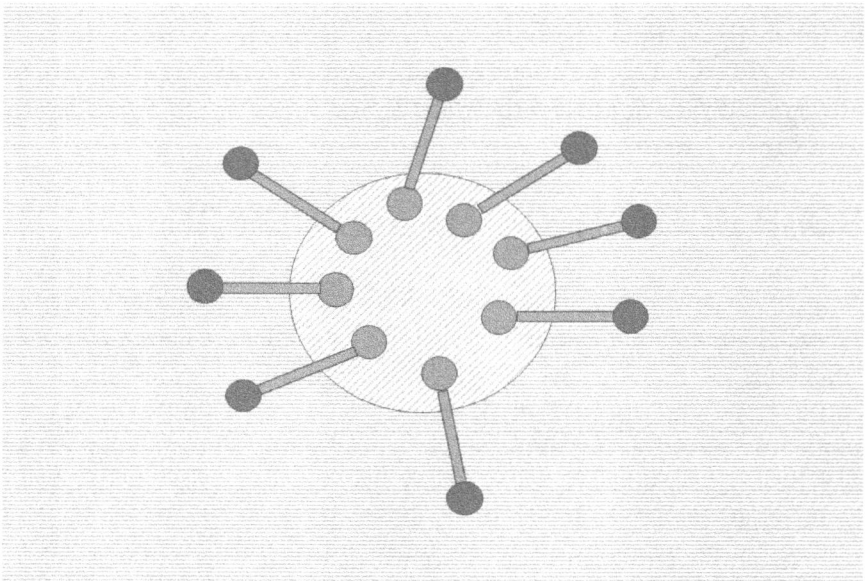

Figure 13.2 Surfactant molecules embedding in an oil/grease droplet.

Because of this action, when one washes with soap, the hydrophilic end of the surfactant molecule projects out into the surrounding water and, in effect, lowers the surface tension of the water. Agitation creates foam which emulsifies the oil and grease globules on the skin so that they, together with any dirt particles, can be washed away with water.

SOAP SURFACTANTS

Soap is made by the reaction of fats or oils, known as triglycerides[69], with a base or alkali such as sodium hydroxide (lye[70]) or potassium hydroxide (potash). This interaction, known as *saponification*, yields soap surfactants and glycerol (glycerin), the latter being used in a variety of other products or may be left in the soap as a softening agent. The commonest soap surfactant is sodium stearate although, depending on the fat being used, a variety of other chemical compounds (surfactants) are produced. When the base that is used to interact with the triglycerides is potassium hydroxide, the reaction product is liquid soap whereas sodium hydroxide produces harder, solid soap.

When one washes in hard water, the sodium (or potassium) stearate reacts with calcium and magnesium in the water to produce insoluble calcium and magnesium stearates – what is known as soap scum.

In contrast to soap, body washes and shower gels mainly use chemicals such as the salts of lauryl sulfates and laureth sulfates as the main surfactants. Other compounds such as cetyl alcohol and glycerol stearate are also present to give the body wash or gel an opaque or pearlescent appearance.

SOAP vs. BODY WASH

Although soap, body wash and shower gel all clean the body through their emulsifying action on oils and grease, their effects on the skin differ because of differences in the pH (or the acidity and alkalinity) of skin and the washing agents.

---

69   The triglycerides (oils and fats) used in making toilet soaps are derived from coconut, olive or palm oils as well as tallow.

70   A lye is a metal hydroxide traditionally obtained by leaching ashes, or is the name given to a strong alkali that is soluble in water and produces a caustic or high pH solution. "Lye" is a commonly-used name for sodium hydroxide although, historically, it was applied to potassium hydroxide and, in fact, the term "lye" actually refers to any member of a wide range of metal hydroxides.

The pH of skin is slightly acidic, commonly ranging from 4.5 to 5.5, compared to that for pure water which is neutral with a pH of 7. In contrast, soap tends to be relatively alkaline with a pH ranging from 8.0 to 11.0 whereas the pH of body washes and shower gels is usually in the range of 4.0 to 6.0. So, body wash and shower gel have pH values closer to that of skin and, consequently, do not have the drying effect on the skin often found with soap.

Soaps, body washes and shower gels usually also contain various other additives designed to increase consumer appeal and, often, to achieve specific effects. Certain additives may be used to improve hydration of the skin, particularly with soaps. The soaps/gels may also contain emollient or skin-softening agents and even anti-bacterials to remove body odor and/or microbes on the skin. Perfumes and essential oils are common additives to soaps, shower gels and body washes to impart a pleasing scent as well as to take advantage of the effect of the essential oils on the skin and the senses. Interestingly, Young Living markets Bath & Shower Gel Base, a gel base that allows the consumer to add a few drops of their favorite essential oil or oil blend to create a luxurious custom bath or shower gel.

ESSENTIAL OILS and SKIN CONDITIONS

Many essential oils are used in cosmetic preparations because they are natural and have low mammalian toxicity. The applications in cosmetics and skin care include treating dryness, providing skin protection, emollient (softening) action, anti-aging and skin toning, anti-inflammatory effects, antimicrobial activity, free-radical scavenging and to treat acne and psoriasis. A major benefit of essential oils in cosmetics is that they not only impart a pleasant aroma, provide emollience and improve skin elasticity but add shine and conditioning effects in hair care products. Some important applications of EOs in skin care are discussed below.

TIGHTENING SAGGY SKIN

Loose or saggy skin is a widespread naturally-occurring problem for women (and men) that has many different causes. Commonly, it is the result of aging but also from losing fat or after childbirth.

Although loose skin is almost inevitable for humans, it can be firmed up with essential oils which can be used on skin as anti-aging and pore-reducing treatments. The best essential oils for this are:

Almond oil

Almond oil has a high vitamin E content so that it is an excellent moisturizer. It also helps tighten skin (and remove stretch marks!) and through its anti-oxidative properties, it will help repair and rejuvenate skin cells.

Frankincense oil

Frankincense oil can improve the appearance of saggy skin, help correct and remove age and sun spots. It has a protective effect on the skin, safeguarding it from blemishes, large pores and reducing wrinkles. Research indicates that frankincense oil assists resolution of scars, helps wound healing and has a "lifting" effect on skin. It can be used directly but is best used with a carrier oil.

Neroli Oil

Neroli oil has a high citral[71] content which helps regenerate the skin by stimulating the growth of new tissue cells while repairing old cells. It can be applied directly to the skin or blended with carriers like glycerin or vitamin E oil for extra moisturizing effects.

These three essential oils are very potent and although almond oil can be used undiluted, blending neroli and frankincense oils with carrier oils might be advisable, especially for those with sensitive skins.

---

71 *Citral* is a pale yellow, water-insoluble liquid with a strong lemony odor, usually obtained from the oils of lemon and orange.

In particular, users must bear in mind that it is possible for any highly potent essential oils to cause skin irritation and inflammation, sun-sensitivity and allergic reactions when used undiluted. Consequently, pregnant women and nursing mothers, and those with dermatological and medical conditions, should seek the advice of a dermatologist, healthcare provider or certified aromatherapist before using any essential oils on the skin.

TREATING ACNE

Acne vulgaris, commonly known as *acne*, is a chronic and sometimes severe skin disorder that occurs when hair follicles are clogged with dead skin cells and oil from the skin. It is characterized by blackheads, whiteheads, pimples, oily skin and sometimes scarring and cysts. This disorder affects about 80-90% of adolescents and some 50% of adults over 20 years of age in the Western World, and is estimated to affect 633 million people worldwide, making it the 8th most common disease afflicting man.

Although acne is generally less common in adulthood, it can persist in about half of affected adolescents into their twenties and thirties, and sometimes into their forties. In fact, acne probably accounts for at least 40% of all patient visits to dermatologists.

Acne primarily affects areas of the skin with a relatively high number of oil glands, such as the face, upper part of the chest or what is commonly called the décolletage, and the back. Genetics is thought to be the primary cause of acne in 80% of cases and neither cleanliness nor sunlight exposure are considered to be causative elements in the disorder. Another factor in acne is the increase in hormones such as testosterone that occurs during puberty for both sexes. Finally, another frequent factor in acne is excessive growth of several bacteria normally present on the skin, notably *Propionibacterium acnes* and *Staphylococcus epidermidis* as well as several other bacterial species that are present in lesser amounts.

Treatment options for acne include lifestyle changes, reduced carbohydrate intake (notably sugar), medications, and medical procedures. Treatments applied directly to the affected skin include azelaic acid[72], benzoyl peroxide, salicylic acid and retinoids. Hormone treatments are often advocated for acne treatment and, apparently, several types of birth control pills help against acne in women. Topical and oral antibiotics may also be used and at one time, tetracycline was extensively prescribed as an acne treatment. However, the development of antimicrobial resistance by both *Propionibacterium acnes* and *Staphylococcus epidermidis*, and other dermal bacteria, has reduced antibiotic effectiveness. Because acne can often be refractory, growing antibiotic resistance and the understandable reluctance of women to undergo hormonal therapy, there is a growing need for alternative and safe therapies to treat the condition.

Despite the well-recognized antimicrobial capabilities of essential oils (see Chapters 4 and 5), there have been relatively few studies on their use in treating acne. Most attention has been paid to evaluating the usefulness of tea tree oil (Melaleuca alternifolia) in treating acne. In fact, several clinical reports indicate that both topical 5% tea tree oil and a tea tree oil gel are effective treatments for mild to moderate acne vulgaris. The beneficial effect of tea tree oil (TTO) has been ascribed to its main constituent, terpinen-4-ol, because it is a potent anti-inflammatory agent. Interestingly, there has been at least one report that cedarwood oil was helpful in controlling acne.

Although there has been no systematic assessment of CAM therapies in treating skin conditions such as acne, there is growing interest in using essential oils and, particularly, oil blends for this purpose. Because the chemistry and flora of skin are so complex, taking advantage of the potential synergistic effects with essential oil blends may be an exciting and effective approach to treating acne.

TREATNG PSORIASIS

Psoriasis is a chronic autoimmune disease affecting 2-4% of the population that is characterized by patches of skin that are typically red,

---

72   Azelaic acid is a dicarboxylic acid used to treat the pimples and swelling caused by acne. Its action in treating acne is by killing the bacteria that infect pores and decreasing the production of keratin, the protein that protects epithelial cells from damage, but which has the potential to kill the cell and can lead to the development of acne.

dry, itchy and scaly. Psoriasis can vary in severity from small, local-ized patches to complete body coverage; injury to the skin patches can trigger psoriatic skin changes at that spot. There are five main types of psoriasis: plaque, guttate, inverse, pustular and erythrodermic; of these, plaque psoriasis, also known as *psoriasis vulgaris*, makes up about 90% of cases. The typical appearance of plaque psoriasis is red patches with white scales on the uppermost surface with the most commonly affected areas of the body being the back of the forearms, shins, the navel area, and the scalp. Psoriasis has been associated with an increased risk of depression, lymphomas, cardiovascular disease, Crohn's disease and psoriatic arthritis, the latter affecting up to 30% percent of sufferers.

Psoriasis is generally thought to be a genetic disease triggered by environmental factors. The symptoms may worsen during winter and can be exacerbated by certain medications, such as beta-blockers and NSAIDs[73], as well as psychological stress and infections. Apparently, the underlying mechanism for the disease is a reaction of the immune system to skin cells. Men and women are affected with equal frequency and although the disease may begin at any age, it typically starts in adulthood.

There is no cure for psoriasis but the symptoms can be controlled, to a greater or lesser degree, by treatments such as topical salicylic acid, topical steroids, ultraviolet light, oral retinoids (forms of vitamin A) such as acitretin, immune system suppressants (e.g. methotrexate and cyclosporine) and some very newly-approved medications (known as immunomodulator drugs) that work with the immune system to decrease the body's response to inflammation. Unfortunately, many of these medications are expensive and may have quite severe side-effects so that sufferers often opt for alternative treatments.

---

73 *Beta blockers* (also known as β-blockers and beta-adrenergic blocking agents) are drugs used to reduce blood pressure and work by blocking the effects of the hormone epinephrine (adrenaline). NSAIDs are nonsteroidal anti-inflammatory drugs and are used to reduce pain, lower fever, prevent blood clots and, at higher doses, to decrease inflammation.

Carrier Oils in Psoriasis Treatment

Essential oils are increasingly being studied for the tropical treatment for psoriasis. However, pure (100%) oils, as stated many times within this book, are concentrated and very potent, and should be diluted with a carrier oil. Carrier oils are discussed below and in Chapter 16.

The commonly used carrier, coconut oil, is not an essential oil but it does have anti-inflammatory properties that may help ease psoriasis pain and discomfort. Because the oil moisturizes the skin and scales, it is often recommended as a treatment for scalp psoriasis. Not only that, coconut oil typically does not cause any side-effects or other interactions with the body and is used routinely in cooking. Further, because coconut oil contains lauric acid, it may help block penetration of the skin by bacteria and viruses.

Like coconut oil, castor oil is not an essential oil but is used as a carrier or vehicle for applying essential oil. Castor oil is a natural emollient and anecdotal accounts suggest that daily use may speed up healing and moisturize areas of dry, flaky skin as well as help remove skin toxins. However, it should be noted that many commercially available castor oils may have been manufactured through chemical processing or were extracted from pesticide-treated seeds. Checking the labelling may avoid potential side-effects like skin irritation and, regardless of its source, castor oil is not recommended for women who are pregnant or breastfeeding.

Argan oil also is used as a carrier oil and rarely elicits any allergic reactions. The high vitamin E content of the oil makes it a good skin hydrator as well as possibly helping skin metabolism, reducing inflammation and providing protection against the sun. Because argan oil is both anti-inflammatory and antiseptic, it can be useful in psoriasis by reducing dryness, redness, swelling and itchiness. It should be noted that argan oils may be used in cosmetics (typically in hair care and skin care products) and for culinary purposes but the two types of oils, i.e. cosmetic and culinary, are produced differently and should not be confused. Bottle labels should be checked to ensure that cosmetic argan oil is not ingested by mistake.

Essential Oils for Psoriasis

Essential oils have been used for thousands of years in aromatherapy, massage therapy and in many CAM therapies for numerous health issues, including skin conditions like psoriasis. However, until comparatively recently, there have been few scientific studies regarding the use of essential oils as a psoriasis treatment and most of the available information on this application of EOs is anecdotal. The expert consensus appears to be that essential oils should not be a primary or first-line treatment option for psoriasis, rather that they are best used as a complementary therapy to a regular or standard treatment regimen.

Notwithstanding the above comment, more scientifically validated information is becoming available regarding the use of essential oils in psoriasis treatment. Interestingly, there has been one study that indicates aromatherapy may be an alternative management approach to psoriasis. Another recent study evaluated the clinical pharmacology of bergamot (*Citrus bergamia*) essential oil (BEO) as reported in several different articles. A detailed analysis of these various scientific articles indicated that BEO aromatherapy could be safe and useful to reduce stress symptoms and one study suggested a potential supportive role in ultraviolet B light therapy against psoriasis. Overall, it was concluded that many studies on BEO were of low quality and the effectiveness and safety of this oil cannot be regarded as definitive. So, the consensus opinion is that aromatherapy has both physiological and psychological benefits for psoriasis sufferers. The effectiveness of aromatherapy for psoriatics presumably comes from its stress-reducing benefits, stress and depression being amongst the contributing factors to psoriasis flare-ups.

At least two scientific articles report studies on tea tree oil (TTO) in the treatment of psoriasis, the premise being that the anti-bacterial, antiviral, anti-inflammatory and antifungal properties of the oil may be beneficial in treating the skin patches. The initial findings of these studies certainly show promise, and numerous anecdotal comments indicate that topical TTO does reduce redness and itching in psoriasis.

Most anecdotal reports on the use of EOs for psoriasis center around lavender, peppermint, geranium and black cumin seed oils. Lavender oil, probably the most studied of any essential oil, has been recommended in aromatherapy for stress relief, relaxation, headaches and, notably, to alleviate the emotional "triggers" of psoriasis. Because lavender possesses antibacterial and antifungal properties, it is also recommended for the treatment of abrasions and minor wounds and burns. In addition, lavender has also been suggested as an antipruritic (anti-itch) agent to inhibit the itching associated with various skin conditions. The latter include sunburn, allergic reactions, contact dermatitis, eczema, psoriasis, fungal infections, insect bites and urticaria (skin rashes) caused by plants such as poison ivy, poison oak and stinging nettles. However, pregnant and breast-feeding women, as well as diabetics, are advised to avoid using lavender oil, especially when undiluted. Further, topical overuse of this oil may result in nausea, vomiting, or headaches in susceptible individuals.

Geranium oil is believed to have a stress-relieving effect and that its use will improve circulation and reduce inflammation. It is also thought to promote the growth and regeneration of healthy skin cells. However, because geranium oil can slow or stop blood flow, sufferers from high blood pressure and those at risk of cardiovascular disease should be cautious in their use of this oil. When used to treat psoriasis, acne or dermatitis, geranium oil should be diluted with a carrier oil like coconut, castor or argan oil. There appear to be no valid scientific evaluations of germanium oil in treating acne or psoriasis.

Peppermint oil may help alleviate any itching and pain around psoriasis patches. At least 25 different species of peppermint plant with over 600 varieties are known but, regardless of the specific source of the peppermint oil, the principal and most important constituent of the oil(s) is the menthol content. It is this menthol content that is effective in treating pruritis (itching) due to psoriasis, scabies and even herpes blisters. Commonly, peppermint oil is added to water in a spray bottle and spritzed onto the affected areas of skin. In small doses, peppermint rarely causes any side-effects, but occasional allergic reactions have been observed.

Black cumin seed oil (commonly known as *black seed oil*) is reputed to have anti-inflammatory, anti-bacterial and antifungal properties and it is used in animals (and humans) for its anthelmintic[74]

---

74 *Anthelmintics* or antihelminthics are antiparasitic drugs that expel parasitic worms and other internal parasites from the body but without causing damage to the host.

properties. Used topically, black seed oil will help reduce inflammation while promoting or speeding up the skin's healing processes. It is also considered to be an excellent moisturizer and when used in psoriasis, it is claimed to reduce scale thickness. However, black seed oil may slow blood clotting and lower blood pressure, therefore it may not be recommended for people with low blood pressure, blood clotting disorders, patients on blood thinners or for diabetics. Likewise, it may not be advisable for use by pregnant women. An interesting corollary with black seed oil is that it is claimed to have a sedative effect.

FINAL THOUGHTS

It should be obvious from this chapter and from the discussion in other chapters of this book that essential oils have an important role in skin care. This not only includes cosmetics together with hair and skin care products but also in their topical action in treating acne and psoriasis. However, despite being natural products, essential oils can be very potent agents when used as primary treatments or as adjuncts in other therapeutic approaches. For this reason, it is often advisable to regard essential oils as medications and, therefore, they should be used with care, especially when used undiluted or if ingested. In most instances, essential oils are generally not recommended for pregnant or breast-feeding women and, it should be noted, some oils may interact with certain medications or have an adverse effect on some health issues. Further, although allergic reactions to essential oils are uncommon, when used undiluted or on sensitive skin, they can cause irritation and other adverse effects.

Because some essential oils can have a desquamatous effect[75], it is always advisable to consult a dermatologist or healthcare provider before using any essential oil as an adjunct to current or projected treatment for psoriasis or acne. Further, it is always important that any essential oil be thoroughly researched before use since each oil carries its own cautions and potential interactions. Also, users should be cau-

---

75 *Desquamation* (also called skin peeling) is the shedding of the outermost membrane or layer of a tissue, such as the skin. Desquamation is how salicylic acid removes warts from the skin through its irritant effect.

tious in their selection of essential oils because, as stated in this book, many so-called EOs are not natural or pure.

The scientific literature on the role of essential oils in treating skin disease is growing, but much of what is available is viewed as being questionable by experts in the field, often because of poor study design, inadequate controls or simply misleading data. Nevertheless, there is a mounting body of scientific information, and not just anecdotal comments, indicating that essential oils have a valuable role to play in treating skin diseases, a role that will inevitably widen as further research is undertaken.

CHAPTER 14

HALITOSIS

Halitosis, the medical term for oral malodor or, simply, bad breath, is a <u>symptom</u> giving those afflicted by the condition a noticeably unpleasant <u>breath</u> <u>odor</u>. The worldwide prevalence of halitosis is estimated to be in the range of 22-50%[76] and it appears to become more common as people age. Curiously, halitosis is one condition that affects others more than the actual sufferer but when the latter becomes aware of having bad breath, it often leads to anxiety, self-consciousness and sometimes to depression, obsessive compulsive disorder (OCD) and social isolation. This is often because bad breath is widely viewed as a social taboo and affected people may be stigmatized. One consequence of this stigmatization is that over $1 billion per year is estimated to be spent on mouthwashes, breath mints and other approaches to halitosis in the United States alone. However, it should be mentioned that there is also a significant prevalence of non-genuine halitosis when "sufferers" feel or sense that they have bad breath, but which is undetected by others. In such cases, counselling may be helpful for those convinced they have bad breath despite assurances to the contrary from others.

As discussed later in this chapter, people with poor oral hygiene and periodontal conditions often suffer from oral malodor and

---

76 Akaji EA, Folaranmi N, Ashiwaju O. Halitosis: a review of the literature on its prevalence, impact and control. Oral Health Prev. Dent. (2014) 12(4):297-304.

although uncommon, certain medical conditions such as ketoacidosis or liver failure also can result in halitosis. Gastroesophageal reflux disease (GERD) or simply indigestion and acid reflux is also a frequent cause of bad breath. Notwithstanding these comments, halitosis has two primary causes for the average sufferer, notably exogenous[77] sources and oral bacteria.

DIET AND HALITOSIS

Diet intake is probably the commonest cause of *transient* bad breath and although food-induced halitosis can last for several hours after eating or drinking. Transient halitosis is common after consuming what are termed volatile or odiferous[78] foodstuffs, notably spicy or pungent foods such as curries, garlic and onions. Apparently, the Asian fruit durian, known as both the king of fruits and the smelliest fruit in the world, is claimed to produce the most severe transient oral malodor. Other notable causes of transient halitosis include smoking and drinking beer, wine and other alcoholic beverages as well as coffee, as discussed later.

Food-related bad breath results from particles of volatile foods becoming trapped between the teeth, in the dental sulci, on the cheeks and tongue as well as beneath and towards the back of the tongue. Obviously, the way to reduce and possibly eliminate food-derived malodor is by avoiding odiferous foods but, unfortunately, many cuisines rely on volatile (i.e. malodor-causing) spices to flavor foods and impart their distinctive tastes.

Alcohol-containing Beverages

Pungent beverages such as wine, beer, liquors and even coffee can also cause transient halitosis, and many is the motorist that has been breathalyzed because the police officer could smell alcohol on the breath. Alcoholic beverage-induced halitosis is actually quite a complex process. The body treats alcohol as a toxin and does not absorb it; instead,

---

77 Exogenous means coming from or produced outside the body.

78 Anything that is *odoriferous* carries a smell, the word being made up of *odor* or smell and the Latin word *ferre* meaning "to carry."

alcohol is slowly metabolized by the liver. However, until the alcohol is completely metabolized, it stays in the bloodstream and therefore enters the lungs, the latter effect, in turn, imparting a distinct smell to the breath.

Consumption of alcoholic beverages often disrupts the oral biome, the balance of good *vs.* bad bacteria in the mouth, usually inducing a higher concentration of "bad" bacteria. This, in turn, increases the risk not only of gum disease and tooth decay, but also of systemic effects such as cancer and heart disease. Another effect of drinking alcohol is that it can trigger gastric acid reflux, which causes odiferous stomach acid to creep up into the throat and taint the breath.

Alcohol also can cause dry mouth which may have a variety of effects on the oral cavity and the body. Finally, as most people are aware, alcohol-containing beverages have a diuretic effect due to the way the body metabolizes alcohol. This diuresis[79] causes excess urination, dehydration and morning dry-mouth after alcohol consumption the previous evening. Unfortunately, drinking water with alcoholic-containing beverages does not ward off dehydration or prevent "hang-overs".

Other causes of halitosis

Smoking and tobacco products also cause oral malodor due to the deposition of fine particulate matter on the teeth, gums and tongue as well as the skin around the mouth. Not only that, tobacco residues can cause dry mouth together with disruption of the oral biome. The latter effect can be a source of halitosis as well as lead to gingivitis.

Mild transient oral malodor, commonly known as "morning breath", often arises during sleep. Morning breath occurs most often with people with nasal obstructions due to upper respiratory tract and sinus infections, but it can also be the result of sleeping in a hot, dry atmosphere which can dry out the oral cavity and nasal airways. Mouth breathers and those wearing oral appliances such as bite guards or dentures during sleep likewise may experience morning breath.

---

79 *Diuresis* is when the body has an excess of certain substances in the fluid filtered through the kidneys. This fluid eventually becomes urine and increases the amount of water expelled by the body, leading to increased or excessive urination.

Dry mouth syndrome

Sufferers from dry mouth or *xerostomia* tend to be more prone to halitosis than those with a normal salivary flow. There are many causes of dry mouth, Table 14.1, but especially mouth breathers and sufferers from blocked nasal passages.

Alcohol consumption
Allergies/congestion
Autoimmune disorders like lupus and Sjögren's Syndrome
Caffeinated beverages (coffee, tea)
Chronic sinusitis and post-nasal drip
Cold/allergy medications
Dysfunctional saliva glands
Medications such as antidepressants and hypertensives
Smoking

Table 14.1 Potential causes of dry mouth

The reason why dry mouth syndrome often exacerbates halitosis is because it creates a less-aerated environment that is conducive to bacterial proliferation, notably anaerobic bacteria as discussed below (see also Appendix F). Not only that, when someone predominantly breathes through the mouth, e.g. because of sinus problems or a cold, saliva flow in the mouth is decreased, i.e. patients have a "dry mouth". This has a two-fold effect, namely depriving the oral cavity of the flow of oxygenated saliva with its natural anti-bacterial action but also reducing the mouth's ability to naturally sluice away food particles by saliva throughout the oral cavity.

Another aspect of xerostomia is that the pH of saliva drops (i.e., it becomes more acidic), exacerbating dental decay and stimulating proliferation of Gram-negative bacteria and, consequently, chronic halitosis. A comparable effect is often found with people that engage in intense diets that restrict caloric intake. Limited caloric intake restricts the supply of food-derived glycogen[80] to the liver which leads to a diminished supply of energy to the body and then to ketosis[81]. Ketosis produces ketones that infiltrate the bloodstream and lowers the pH of blood and saliva, allowing greater growth of anaerobic bacteria in the acidic, drier and reduced aerated conditions of the oral cavity.

Untreated dry mouth syndrome intensifies the development of tooth and gum diseases which, in turn, may lead to more serious conditions such as periodontitis, tooth loss, sepsis and infections of the jaws or the neck. Even when good oral hygiene is practiced, poor salivary flow and lack of aeration can still lead to serious dental and systemic health problems.

Sinusitis and post-nasal drip

Sinusitis and post-nasal drip frequently contribute to halitosis because the mucus that accumulates in the back of the throat and on the tongue's dorsal (upper) surface is rich in proteins, and these constitute a food supply for anaerobic bacteria. The metabolic processes involved in microbial digestion of mucus can release copious amounts of sulfurous, smelly compounds within the mouth. In fact, up to about 15% of halitosis cases may be ascribed to disorders and/or infections in the nasal cavity, the sinuses and the throat.

Oral malodor can also be sourced from the lungs and, for example, bronchitis which is often an infection resulting from progression of sinus infections, has a distinct and unpleasant malodor.

Dentures and Oral Appliances

Many complete and partial denture wearers have halitosis, commonly because of microbial infestation of the pink plastic (acrylic resin) of the denture. Unfortunately, a high proportion of denture wearers may be unaware of their halitosis, possibly contributing to the statement that

---

80 *Glycogen* is a polysaccharide deposited in bodily tissues as a store of carbohydrates. When hydrolyzed. glycogen forms glucose, an energy source for the body.

81 *Ketosis* is a metabolic state characterized by raised levels of ketones in the body tissue. Ketosis is often a typical pathology with diabetes, or it may be the result of a diet that is very low in carbohydrates.

bad breath afflicts older patients more than younger people if only because a greater proportion of the elderly have dentures.

Plaque, food residues and microbial build-up on dentures will be a continuing source of oral malodor. This is because the surface of the acrylic resin (the pink "gum work" of the denture) is covered in microscopic voids and porosities which act as reservoirs or wells for considerable numbers of bacterial and fungal species.

In fact, the array of bacterial species that can inhabit dentures[82,83] is astonishing, and many of them lead to significant oral and systemic health problems if uncontrolled. So, not only do these bacteria and fungi cause health issues, they markedly contribute to halitosis. Other resin-based (plastic) oral appliances such as bite guards and mouthguards have the same issue regarding microbial proliferation and wearers likewise can suffer from halitosis as well as other conditions.

Although many of these bacterial-induced problems can be reduced by careful and regular cleaning of the denture, complete removal can be very difficult and requires effort. Brushing all surfaces with anti-bacterial soap, immersion in a bath of effervescent cleanser, avoiding wearing the appliance continuously and brushing regularly with such products as Thieves toothpaste and mouthwash can both freshen the appliance surface and reduce or remove bacteria.

Halitosis and Oral Bacteria

Most cases of halitosis (85-90%), originate within the oral cavity[84] and the term "oral malodor" is appropriate. In fact, concern over bad breath is the 3rd most common reason, after tooth decay and gum disease, that people seek dental care. Although oral malodor can affect

---

82   Glass R.T., Bullard J. W., Hadley C. S. et al. Partial spectrum of microorganisms found in dentures and possible disease implications. J. Am Osteo Ass (2001) 101: 92-94. Glass R. T., Wood C. R. Bullard J. W. et al. General Dentistry (2007) 55: 436-440.

83   von Fraunhofer J. A. and Loewy Z. G. Factors involved in microbial colonization of oral prosthetics. General Dentistry (2009) 57: 136-143.

84   De Geest S, Laleman I, Teughels W, et al. Periodontal diseases as a source of halitosis: a review of the evidence and treatment approaches for dentists and dental hygienists. Periodontol 2000 (2016) 71(1):213-27.

healthy individuals, it is more prevalent in those with poor oral hygiene and concomitant tooth decay, gingivitis and periodontitis. Adult periodontitis caused by the gradual but progressive loss of the periodontal attachment to the teeth, will cause varying degrees of oral malodor which intensifies as the periodontitis progresses.

In this context, a very recent scientific study[85] identified *Porphyromonas gingivalis,* the principal pathogen in chronic periodontitis, together with neurotoxic proteases from the bacterium called *gingipains* in the brain of Alzheimer's disease patients. The study went on to report that small-molecule inhibitors targeting gingipains blocked *P. gingivalis* brain colonization in mice. The study data suggest that gingipain inhibitors could be valuable for treating *P. gingivalis* brain colonization and neurodegeneration in Alzheimer's disease. This study clearly suggests that gum disease, notably chronic periodontitis, can not only cause halitosis but other even more serious conditions.

Although over 500 species of bacteria inhabit the oral cavity[86], it appears that anaerobic Gram-negative bacteria[87], the species that are found in nearly all dental infections including abscesses, dental plaque, gingivitis, periodontitis and pulpitis (inflammation of dental pulp) are those most commonly associated with bad breath[88]. However, it is possible that some types of Gram-positive oral bacteria, notably streptococci, may also contribute to VSC formation.

In simple terms, oral malodor can be caused by microbial degradation of both non-sulfur and sulfur-containing amino acids from

---

85   Dominy S.S, Lynch, C, Ermini F, *et al. Porphyromonas gingivalis* in Alzheimer's disease brains: Evidence for disease causation and treatment with small-molecule inhibitors. Science Advances (2019) Jan 23, vol. 5, no. 1, eaau3333 (DOI: 10.1126/sciadv.aau3333).

86   The bacteria typically associated with dental plaque build-up around teeth are *Fusobacterium nucleatum, Porphyromonas gingivalis, Tannerella forsythia, Prevotella intermedia* and *Porphyromonas endodontalis.* However, the bacteria most involved in the build-up of debris on the dorsal (upper) surface of the tongue are *Veillonella, Actinomyces, Prevotella, Capnocytophaga* and *Odontomyces,* the latter generally found in people 70+ years of age.

87   See Chapter 17 and Appendix F regarding the different types of bacteria and their characteristics.

88   *Treponema denticola, Porphyromonas gingivalis, Tannerella forsythensis, Porphyromonas endodontalis, Prevotella intermedia* and *Eubacterium.*

food residues into bad-smelling gases. These gases, known as volatile sulfur compounds (VSC) include those indicated in Table 14.2 and their names alone are indicative of their pungency.

Methyl mercaptan
Dimethyl sulfide
Hydrogen sulfide
Isovaleric acid
Cadaverine
Skatole
Putrescine

Table 14.2 Volatile organo-sulfur compounds released by bacterial decomposition of food stuffs.

When one or more of these VSC are generated by bacterial action, the released odors are commonly compared to the smell of boiled cabbage, rotten eggs, rancid dairy products and even decaying flesh. It is also known that some of these volatile organic compounds increase patient susceptibility to periodontitis, exacerbating the halitosis.

Although it is not readily apparent, the surfaces of the tongue are relatively rough due to the taste buds and the presence of almost microscopic fissures, recesses and pits. Consequently, bacteria can accumulate and proliferate within these "cavities", particularly towards the back of the tongue where conditions tend to be less clean and relatively dry. With continued growth of bacteria on the tongue, a grayish-white furry coating will form that is comprised of food particles, mucus and sloughed-off epithelial cells. This coating, commonly seen and felt in the morning and by dry mouth sufferers, is a bacterial matrix which will emit noxious fumes, i.e. oral malodor, as proteins within the coating matrix are digested by the bacteria.

Oral thrush

Oral thrush or *candidiasis*[89,90], manifested as white lesions on the tongue and elsewhere in the mouth, can also be a cause of oral malodor. Although oral thrush can affect anyone, it is more likely to occur in babies and older adults. It will also occur in people with suppressed immune systems due to certain health conditions such as uncontrolled diabetes and with people taking medications like prednisone and inhaled corticosteroids as well as antibiotics which upset the body's normal bacterial symbiosis.

Oral thrush is a minor problem for healthy individuals but in people with a weakened immune system, it can lead to more severe symptoms that may be more difficult to control. Interestingly, thrush and concomitant oral malodor often accompany sinus infections.

Candidal infestation of complete (and partial) dentures is relatively common but can have severe systemic effects if not treated properly, particularly with older patients. As with the dentate mouth, careful and regular cleansing of all appliances is necessary to prevent candidiasis and bacterial infestation. Although many patients will try to remove candida deposits through tongue scraping, this has little effect because fungal spores buried within the tongue surface are not eliminated.

The accepted approach to oral candidiasis is either rinsing with an antifungal medication such as nystatin oral suspension or taking pills such as fluconazole. Rinsing with fluconazole suspension may be useful for patients with dry mouth or those who have swallowing difficulties caused by oral candidiasis. A clinical study performed several years ago indicated that melaleuca (tea tree oil) oral solution was effective as an alternative regimen for treating oral thrush in AIDS patients with oropharyngeal candidiasis refractory to fluconazole. However, there are indications that twice-daily rinsing with Young Living's Thieves mouthwash, a wholly natural product containing colloidal silver, pep-

---

89 Oral candidiasis or thrush is a condition in which the fungus/yeast *Candida albicans* accumulates on the tongue and lining of the mouth. Candida is a normal organism in the oral cavity but sometimes it can overgrow and cause symptoms.

90 *Candidiasis* in the mouth and throat is also called oropharyngeal candidiasis whereas candidiasis in the esophagus (the tube connecting the throat and stomach) is called esophageal candidiasis or Candida esophagitis.

permint oil and various other essential oils, is beneficial with regard to thrush.

Treatment of Halitosis

Finding the best treatment for bad breath largely depends on the underlying cause. If the halitosis has a dental origin, then dental treatment for tooth decay, periodontal disease as well as good oral hygiene may help alleviate the condition.

Effective toothbrushing, flossing and the use of water irrigating systems to remove food particles and residues from and between the teeth as well as from the gingival sulcus[91] will reduce and usually prevent dental decay and gum disease, and help eliminate halitosis. The treatment should comprise brushing for at least 2 minutes using a toothpaste containing peppermint or other essential oils (e.g. Young Living Aromabright®) to thoroughly clean the teeth followed by careful rinsing. The best remedy, however, is to rinse the mouth or gargle with an alcohol-free mouthwash for 30 to 60 seconds. About 10-12% of the mouthwash will drift towards the back of the mouth and down the throat, helping to eliminate the anaerobic biofilm on the posterior lingual dorsum of the tongue, the area towards the very back of the mouth that cannot be reached by other means.

It should be noted that most over-the-counter mouthwashes contain alcohol and such products may tend to worsen bad breath. Chronic halitosis patients should benefit from using alcohol-free, oxygenating oral hygiene products and natural (essential oil-infused) dentifrices.

Likewise, careful cleaning of all dental appliances, including dentures, bite guards and mouth guards with antibacterial soap or proprietary effervescent oxidizing cleansers will aid in eliminating bacteria and fungus like *Candida albicans* from the oral appliance. This will reduce the risk of dental caries and gum disease and should also help diminish halitosis. Sucking Thieves Lozenges also helps eliminate bad breath, especially halitosis caused by beverages and foodstuffs.

---

91 The gingival sulcus is the space or gap between a tooth and the surrounding gingival (gum) tissue; the word sulcus derives from the Latin word for a groove.

CHAPTER 15

Essential Oils and Sports Medicine

There has been a strong relationship between athletic performance, nutrition and herbal medicine for centuries. Enhancing
athletic performance has been a highly desirable objective of
athletes, sports figures, trainers and coaches since the days of the Ancient
Greeks. Until recently, however, there have been no clearly demonstra-
ble benefits of **natural** approaches to enhanced athletic performance.
This situation has now changed. No-one can dispute the importance
of good nutrition in athletic performance but what is noteworthy is
that interest in correlating herbal medicine with "sports medicine" has
been growing in recent years. Further, this trend has been accompanied
by an increased interest and research into the effects of essential oils
on athletic performance as well as into their other physiological (and
emotional) effects. The latter have been discussed at some length in
previous chapters, but athletic performance was not addressed.

HERBAL SUPPLEMENTS

Herbal products for public consumption come under a special category
of foods that are classified as "dietary supplements" and are regulated
by the Food and Drug Administration (FDA). They are extracted

from the seeds, berries, leaves, flowers, roots and bark of a wide variety of plants and contain varying amounts of phytochemicals[92]. The latter content depends upon the individual plant and the growth, soil and climate conditions as well as the harvesting and extraction processes (see Chapters 2 and 3). These phytochemicals include carotenoids, polyphenols, alkaloids, flavonoids, glycosides, saponins, and lignans, many of which have long been recognized as providing health benefits.

It is known that the use of herbal supplements by athletes (and non-athletes) has markedly increased over the past 10-15 years not only to enhance muscle growth, performance and strength but also to stimulate fat-burning metabolic effects. There are also claims that herbal supplements can stimulate mental activity. It should be noted, however, that some herbal dietary and botanical supplements can be used as source materials in producing illicit drugs and that many supplements have not been proven to be safe or effective under current FDA standards.

Despite these reservations, plants can provide several essential metabolites, including carbohydrates, lipids and nucleic acids and, as discussed in previous chapters, such secondary metabolites as terpenoids, alkaloids and phenolic compounds. It is the biological properties of these secondary metabolites that are so important to health because they provide such benefits as antimicrobial, antiviral, anti-allergic, anti-thrombotic, anti-atherogenic[93], anti-inflammatory, cardio-protective, vasodilatory and other effects. These biological properties are mediated (or brought about) by their antioxidant characteristics and redox properties. In fact, many phytochemicals can neutralize free radicals, scavenge oxygen and decompose peroxides and, thereby, are

---

92 *Phytochemicals* (also known as <u>phytonutrients</u>) are bioactive chemical compounds that occur naturally in plants and which are considered to be beneficial to human health, such as antioxidants. They are responsible for the color and other organoleptic properties, such as the taste and smell of plants and fruits, etc. [Organoleptic properties are those aspects and characteristics of food, drink or other substances that a person can experience through the senses, notably taste, sight, smell and touch]. Although many phytochemicals have biological significance, e.g. carotenoids and flavonoids, not all are essential nutrients.

93 Preventing or inhibiting atherogenesis or the formation of atheromas (plaques) in arteries.

very important in stabilizing oxidative damage by these destructive agents.

In this context, there have been several studies that looked at the role of herbal supplements in reducing exercise-induced oxidative stress in athletes since a reduction in oxidative stress enhances muscle recovery and energy maintenance during intensive exercise. Herbal supplements with high antioxidant components, e.g. caffeine, ephedrine and Ginseng, would appear to be those that enhance muscle performance. It should be mentioned that although there are research reports which indicate that other plants such as ginkgo or the maidenhair tree (*Ginkgo biloba*), artic root (*Rhodiolarosea*), cordyceps mushroom (*Cordyceps sinensis*) and Tribulus Terrestris may benefit muscle growth and strength, other studies indicate that these supplements have no effect on muscle performance.

Readers should be cautioned that many of these research reports claiming improved muscle performance often do not discuss possible side-effects and/or health risks associated with consuming these supplements. It should also be mentioned that differences in the reported findings of various studies on muscle recovery and performance may be because the plant sources of many of these supplements grow wild. Accordingly, as mentioned previously in this chapter and elsewhere in this book, the effectiveness of supplements can vary with the geographic location where the plants grew as well as fluctuate with the harvesting conditions and the extraction method.

It follows from the above that although the effects of herbal supplements on exercise performance may be somewhat inconclusive, investigating the potential role of essential oils in sports medicine is a logical step in complementary and alternative medicine.

ESSENTIAL OILS and SPORTS PERFORMANCE

There have been several recent studies which clearly demonstrated that essential oils can markedly affect sports performance. However, in contrast to advocates of herbal medicine, the beneficial effects came from both inhalation and ingestion. This is clearly a better, safer and more convenient approach to improving athletic performance and certainly better than the use of pharmaceutical agents.

In a recent study[94], 4 groups of rats swam until exhaustion to determine their endurance limits. One group had rested [Control] for 3 days before swimming while a second group of rats [Fatigue] had swum until exhaustion during the same period and were already tired when the test began. The third and fourth groups had also swum but, after swimming, inhaled essential oils for 10 minutes. One group [PEO] inhaled peppermint essential oil while the rats in the 4th group [EOM] inhaled a mixture of 4 essential oils. This mixture comprised equal parts of orange peel oil (*Citrus sinensis*], clove oil (*Syzigium aromaticum)*, peppermint oil (*Mentha piperita*) and rosemary oil (*Rosmarinus officinalis)*. Thereafter further swimming tests were performed together with blood chemistry studies.

The rats that had inhaled peppermint oil after the first swimming session swam for longer than the control and fatigue groups while the rats exposed to the essential oil mixture performed best of all 4 groups, Figure 15.1:

Post-exercise blood chemistry measurements showed that lactic acid and urea build-up occurred in all 4 test groups, but it was lower for rats in the PEO (peppermint oil) group than for the control and fatigue groups while the build-up was least in the EOM (essential oil mixture) rats, Figure 15.2:

---

94   Zhiyue Li, Fengzhi Wu, Haozhen Shao, et al. Does the Fragrance of Essential Oils Alleviate the Fatigue Induced by Exercise? A Biochemical Indicator Test in Rats. Evidence-Based Complementary and Alternative Medicine (2017) Volume 2017, Article ID 5027372.

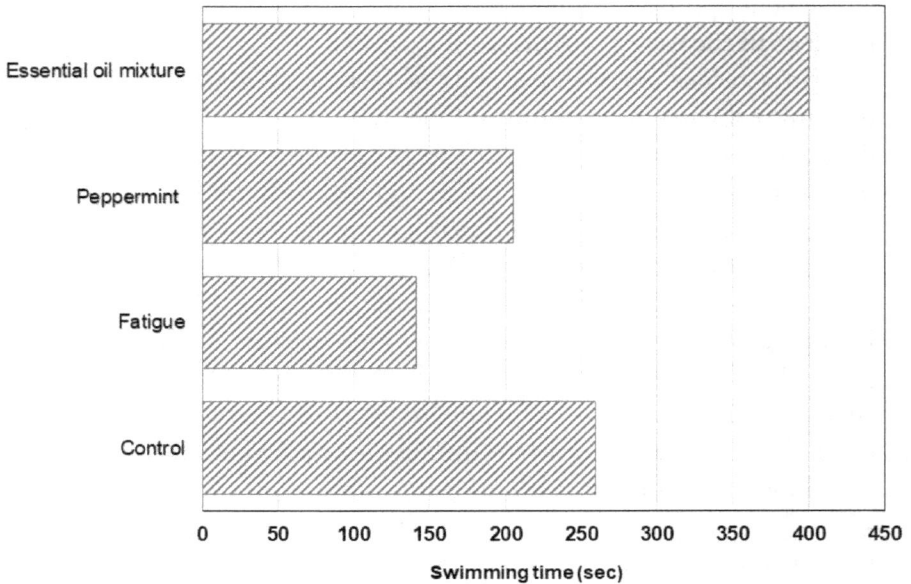

**Figure 15.1 Mean (average) repeat swimming performances
with and without essential oil inhalation.**

The data indicate that whereas lactic acid and urea build-up will occur in the blood after exercise, the inhalation of essential oils markedly reduces this build-up. Further, while peppermint oil is effective, the benefit of the essential oil mixture is considerably greater. Other hematological (blood chemistry) studies showed the essential oil mixture also prevented increase in the concentration of malondialdehyde[95] after the swimming session. At the same time, the essential oil mixture increased the concentration of the detoxifying and antioxidant enzyme glutation-peroxidase which neutralizes free radicals.

---

95 *Malondialdehyde* is a highly reactive organic compound that occurs naturally and is a marker for oxidative stress. It is formed when free radicals attack cell membranes

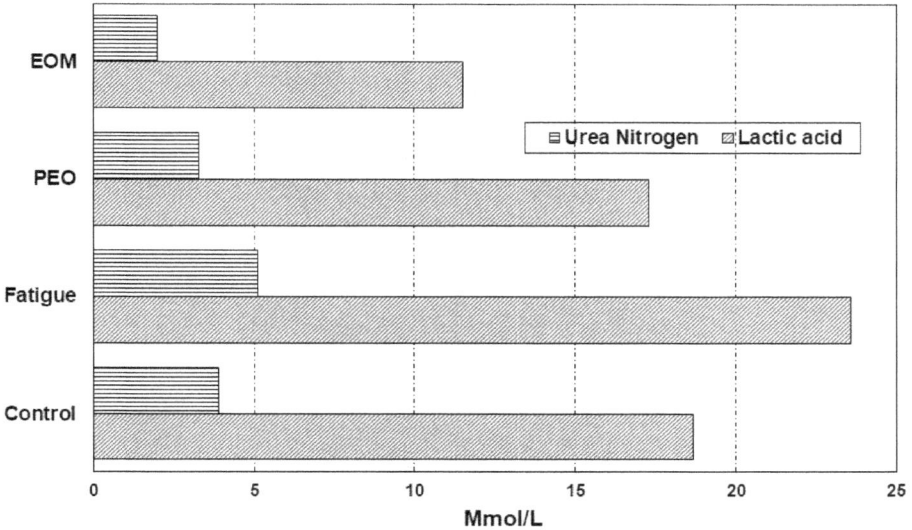

Figure 15.2 Serum build-up of lactic acid and urea after exercise.

The researchers concluded that the inhalation of a mixture of the essential oils of orange, clove, peppermint and rosemary may significantly relieve exercise-induced fatigue. Based on the reduction of the blood urea nitrogen and lactic acid levels, the reported effect was ascribed to the inhibition of the production and accumulation of metabolites. It was also suggested that inhalation of the essential oil mixture protects the cell structure from attack and damage after exercising to exhaustion by the high antioxidant activity of the oil mixture, as shown by the enhanced activity of antioxidant enzymes. The research data suggest that inhalation of essential oils improves the metabolism of the muscle cells and may prevent breakdown of muscle protein. Overall, the findings provide an experimental basis for developing a natural anti-fatigue spray.

Another study investigated the effects of peppermint oil on human exercise performance.[96] Blood pressure and respiratory indices were measured for 12 healthy male students who drank 500 ml of mineral water containing 0.05 ml peppermint oil a day for 10 days. After

---

96   Meamarbashi A. and Rajabi A. The effects of peppermint oil on exercise performance. Journal of the International Society of Sports Nutrition (2013) 10: 15.

a treadmill-based test, it was found that the peppermint oil improved exercise performance based on measurements of blood pressure, gas analysis and respiratory rate. The improved performance was ascribed to relaxation of the bronchial smooth muscles, substantially increased respiratory and ventilation rates, i.e. enhanced lung function, as well as greater brain oxygen concentration and a decrease in blood lactate levels. It was also noted that the peppermint oil significantly increased the time to exhaustion and the distance covered by the test subjects on the treadmill.

Overall, the described effects are not fully understood. However, various theories were advanced to account for the observed increased performance due to peppermint. These theories included an effect on the central nervous system, increased carbohydrate metabolism, lowering of the lung surface tension and improved pulmonary function. Certainly, peppermint does lower heart rate and the systolic blood pressure, and possibly decreases arterial smooth muscle tonicity (i.e. muscle tone).

The above studies showed that consumption of peppermint oil for several days prior to testing improved exercise performance, blood pressure, respiratory rate and spirometry parameters[97]. However, another study evaluated the acute effects of ingesting peppermint oil in water immediately prior to exercise and found no effect on any performance parameters.

Contrary to those findings, another research study[98] showed that placing a few drops (50 μl) of peppermint oil on the tongue before exercise markedly improved exercise performance. Muscle strength parameters for athletes were before administration of peppermint oil, after 5 minutes and then again after 1 hour compared to drinking mineral water, Figure 15.3.

---

97   *Spirometry* or the measuring of breath is the commonest pulmonary function test, measuring lung function, notably the amount (or volume) and/or flow rate of air that can be inhaled and exhaled.

98   Meamarbashi A. Instant effects of peppermint essential oil on the physiological parameters and exercise performance. Avicenna Journal of Phytomedicine (2014) 4: 72-78.

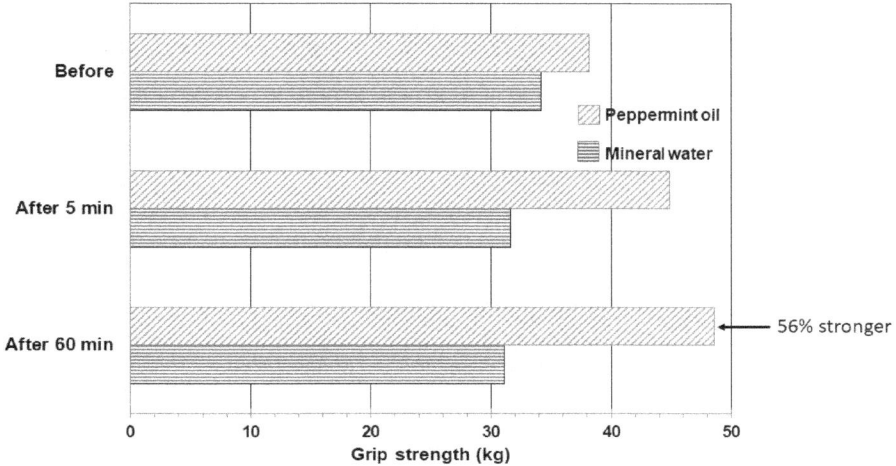

Figure 15.3 Effect of peppermint oil on grip strength.

The performance data showed that the peppermint oil drops increased grip strength quite markedly compared to drinking mineral water. Peppermint oil was also shown to improve performance in standing vertical jumping, standing horizontal jumps as well as in reaction times compared to ingesting mineral water. Interestingly, whereas the peppermint oil drops increased performance, controls that did not receive peppermint oil (i.e. ingested only mineral water) showed either a decrease in strength or minimal change over the test period.

A more recent study[99] looked at the effect of inhalation of orange oil and peppermint oil on lung function and exercise performance. In the study, two groups of 10 young men (physical therapy students) who were fairly closely matched with regard to age, weight, etc., were timed running a distance of 1500 meters. Lung function of each participant was measured with a spirometer. After a 3-day break, one group of participants inhaled orange essential oil and the other peppermint

---

99   Jarad, NA, Al Zabadi H., Rahmal B., et al. The effect of inhalation of *Citrus sinensis* flowers and *Mentha spicata* leave essential oils on lung function and exercise performance: a quasi-experimental uncontrolled before-and-after study. *Journal of the International Society of Sports Nutrition* (2016) 13:36

essential oil. The inhalation regimen comprised nebulizing[100] at a rate of 0.02 ml/kg of body mass mixed with 2 ml of normal saline for 5 min before running 1500 meters.

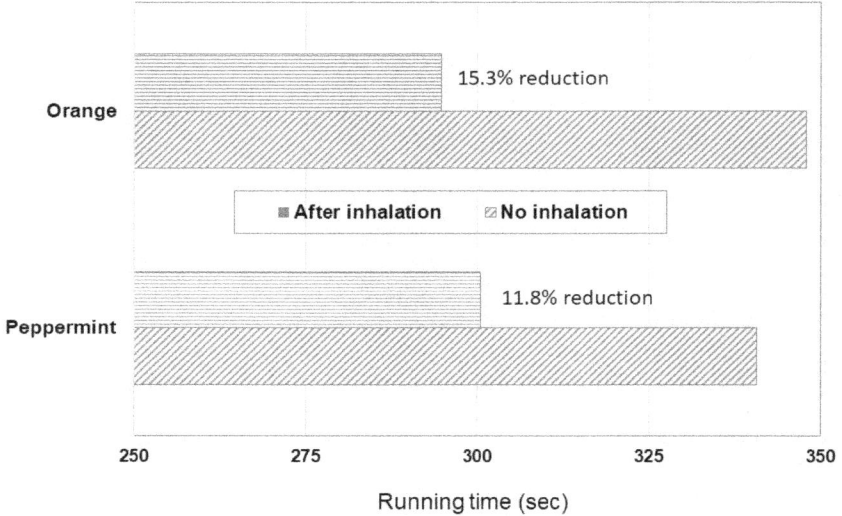

Orange — 15.3% reduction

■ After inhalation   ▨ No inhalation

Peppermint — 11.8% reduction

Running time (sec) — 250, 275, 300, 325, 350

Figure 15.4 Effect of inhaling essential oils on running 1500 meters.

The study showed that inhalation of orange and peppermint oil improved running performance by 15.3 and 11.8% respectively, Figure 15.4. Spirometer measurements likewise showed a significant improvement in lung function for participants after inhalation of the two essential oils. Measurements, for example, of the forced exhalation volume (FEV) showed a significant increase with inhalation of the essential oils. The greater the FEV volume, i.e., the more oxygen the lungs can inhale, obviously provides benefits to athletic performance.

These findings support those of earlier studies which found that inhaling peppermint oil improved running performance under different conditions, and lowered heart rates while running. Likewise, inhaling peppermint can improve aerobic performance and reaction time for athletes. Interestingly, studies have also confirmed that inhalation

---

100   A *nebulizer* is a drug delivery system administering medication in the form of a mist inhaled into the lungs.

of oils from various species of peppermint were effective in reducing muscle pain and fatigue as well as having a muscle relaxation effect. It should be mentioned, however, that there are several different varieties of peppermint plant but the optimal effects on athletic performance are associated with *Mentha piperita.*

At this time, the mechanism for these effects of essential oils are not clear but the collective research data indicate that both ingested and inhaled essential oils benefit athletic performance. What is also interesting is that inhaling both peppermint and orange essential oils appears to be beneficial to lung function, indicating a possible natural approach to relieving the effects of asthma, COPD and other breathing difficulties.

CHAPTER 16

ADVERSE EFFECTS

It goes without saying that almost anything applied to the skin, used to pierce the skin or that is ingested will elicit an adverse effect in at least some percentage of the population. Adverse reactions to tattoos and skin piercing are well-recognized as consequences of subcutaneous dye injections. Some 30% of females (and 3% of males) have allergic reactions such as dermatitis to costume jewelry and many metals, notably to nickel and a few other metals.

In addition to the increasing prevalence of skin problems from tattooing, skin piercing and wearing costume (non-precious metal) jewelry, other localized and systemic hypersensitivity (allergic) reactions appear to be on the rise. Many problems are caused by our surroundings, including such allergens as pollen, pollution, dust mites, pet dander and mold that are pervasive in urban environments. Roughly 20% of the population suffer from one or more of a variety of allergies, notably those caused by cosmetics, foods as well as atmospheric pollutants and environmental factors. Further, a significant proportion of the population is afflicted by autoimmune diseases such as celiac disease (gluten "allergy"), type 1 diabetes, Graves' disease, inflammatory bowel disease (IBS), multiple sclerosis, lupus, psoriasis and rheumatoid arthritis. However, these autoimmune diseases are quite different from allergies although they can mimic the same symptoms. Because both food allergies and autoimmune diseases are relatively common, they can mask adverse reactions to certain potential allergens and be the actual cause of perceived adverse reactions to many products.

There are some 3000 essential oils, many of which are indispensable in industry for the manufacture of fragrances, food flavorants, perfumes and cosmetics. Essential oils such as eucalyptol, menthol, wintergreen (methyl salicylate) and thymol are important ingredients in therapeutic (antiseptic) mouthwashes such as Listerine®. There is also a huge consumer market for essential oils used in aromatherapy and massage therapy as well as other domestic products. Although most essential oils are deemed safe and have been in constant use for literally thousands of years, it is possible that adverse reactions can arise with their use. This is because pure undiluted essential oils are concentrated and, therefore, are highly potent. Further, certain essential oils with their multiplicity of minor ingredients can bind with the proteins in skin and this can cause irritation in sensitive individuals.

On the other hand, given the very large number of EOs and their venerable use by humans, the incidence of allergic reactions to essential oils reported in the scientific literature is astonishingly low when one considers their complex chemistry and multiplicity of components as well as the millions of people exposed to them on a daily basis. The relatively few adverse reactions to essential oils that have been reported in the literature by dermatologists and other healthcare professionals contrasts markedly to that for so many other allergens. That so few verifiable adverse effects to essential oils have been identified is almost totally unexpected in today's health conscious and hypersensitive environment.

SKIN REACTIONS

Many health claims are made for topical treatments with essential oils, including relief of muscle and joint pain, counteracting skin bacterial and fungal infections, treating acne, remedying hair loss and for various digestive and respiratory problems, and to relieve insect bites. Oral use of essential oils also has been shown to have promise for treating certain conditions, notably periodontal (gum) problems, oral thrush and aphthous ulceration (recurrent round or oval sores inside the mouth).

Most of these applications have been discussed in this book and need not be repeated here.

In any discussion of the topical application of essential oils, however, it is important to sound a note of caution. Because of their potency, users should be cautious when topically applying any essential oils to the skin, especially with babies, young children and adults with sensitive skin. Obviously, applying essential oils to broken, burned or irritated skin should be undertaken only by experienced practitioners and healthcare specialists. Not only that, undiluted essential oils should never be applied near mucous membranes such as those in or around the eyes, the nose, the ears, the vagina and anus. Likewise, aromatic gels should never be applied within the nostrils although some practitioners advocate placing a small amount beneath the nostrils to relieve congestion.

According to the American Academy of Dermatology and other professional bodies, perfumes and cosmetics are the leading cause of contact dermatitis (skin irritation). Unfortunately, cutaneous (skin) sensitivity affects more than 2 million people in the USA alone and is on the rise. It is well-known that 100% pure, natural essential oils contain a great many different components, as previously discussed, and many of these can bind with proteins in the skin and may cause skin reactions such as allergic contact dermatitis.

Table 16.1 indicates which essential oils are thought to possibly cause skin irritation from anecdotal reports and a limited number of patch tests. However, there is some controversy over the prevalence of such reactions. For example, essential oils with strong bactericidal properties, e.g., myrrh and tea tree oil, can cause skin irritation (contact dermatitis) when applied directly and undiluted to open wounds and sores. On the other hand, as mentioned in Chapter 4, myrrh has been used to dress severe cuts and battle wounds for thousands of years.

Basil	Orange
Bergamot	Oregano
Camphor	Peppermint
Cassia	Pine
Cinnamon	Rosemary

Citronella	Sandalwood
Clary Sage	Spruce
Clove	Tea Tree (Melaleuca)
Eucalyptus	Thyme
Fir Needle	White Fir
Ginger	Wintergreen
Lemongrass	Ylang Ylang*

Table 16.1 Essential oils that *may* cause skin irritation
(*: Questionable regarding skin irritation)

In contrast to essential oils that may potentially cause irritation, a great many other widely used oils, notably frankincense, lavender, melissa and sandalwood, are generally recognized as less likely to cause sensitivity issues and are often used undiluted. Many essential oil professionals and users also regard melaleuca oil (tea tree oil) and ylang ylang as oils with low irritation potential. There have been, however, a few reports in the scientific literature[101] of adverse reactions such as contact dermatitis caused by tea tree oil and also through exposure to balsam of Peru. Nevertheless, as indicated above, most instances of contact dermatitis appear to be caused by "fragrances", a great many of which are known to contain well-known allergens[102] It should also be mentioned that many skin care products contain vitamin E, also known as tocopherol[65]. Although vitamin E is an important dietary ingredient and its presence in cosmetics might normally be considered to be beneficial, in fact it can cause skin irritation, especially when present in larger amounts.

It should also be mentioned that there are reports in the literature of massage therapists who have experienced occupational contact dermatitis. It is not clear, however, whether the therapists were inherently

---

101 Scientific literature is the term for reports, reviews and other communications (known as "papers"), in (usually) peer-reviewed professional and scientific journals.

102 An *allergen* is a type of antigen (a toxin or other foreign substance) that induces an abnormally strong immune response in the body. Such reactions are known as allergies.

susceptible to skin sensitivity; further, the essential oils or oil blends possibly causing the problem were not identified. Thus, it is unclear whether pure, natural oils caused the perceived problem or whether the contact dermatitis was caused through use of synthetic essential oils. Such skin sensitivity should not be the norm with high quality essential oils for the average (and intermittent) user.

It is possible that repeated and extended use of concentrated oils may cause *scleroderma* or thickening of the skin. On the other hand, the scleroderma is likely also caused by the constant massaging action performed by the therapists, similar effects being found with professional musicians such as piano players as well as stringed instrument players who have to apply pressure with their fingertips to the instruments' keys and metal strings.

Regardless of the absence of any adverse effects on pet owners, transfer of essential oils from their fingers to animals, as mentioned in Chapter 10, should be always be avoided. As a rule, essential oils must never be allowed anywhere near the eyes, noses, ears or anuses of pets. Although tea tree oil has been used as a veterinary antiseptic for many years, veterinary advice should be sought before embarking on essential oil therapy for pets and domestic animals.

Where the essential oils are applied to the skin can also affect the potential responses of patients. The skin on the soles of the feet have larger pores and absorb essential oils more readily than skin elsewhere on the body. Also, some areas of the skin, such as the face and the scalp, are far more sensitive than elsewhere and caution must be exercised when applying essential oils directly and undiluted to these areas.

Carrier Oils (Diluents)

Although contact dermatitis is uncommon, when in doubt, users should dilute the essential oil in a carrier oil and test the diluted oil in a small, inconspicuous area of the patient's skin such as the inside of the forearm to check for irritation and/or sensitivity. If there is no irritation or discomfort within 24-48 hours, then the essential oil or oil blend should be safe to use.

Although many vegetable and seed oils may be used as carriers or diluents for essential oils, most practitioners recommend those listed in

Table 16.2. Some companies such as Young Living market specifically formulated vegetable oil blends as carriers for their pure essential oils.

Almond oil
Aloe Vera oil
Argan oil
Avocado oil
Castor oil
Coconut oil
Fractionated coconut oil
Grapeseed oil
Jojoba oil
Sesame seed oil
Sunflower seed oil
Sweet almond oil

Table 16.2 Suitable carrier oils for Essential Oils

Carrier oils and vegetable oils with a high polyunsaturated fat content, such as fractionated coconut oil[103], are more easily absorbed by the skin than thicker oils like olive oil. Carrier oil mixtures designed specifically for diluting the highly concentrated essential oils before they are applied to individuals are often used by massage therapists when creating their custom massage oils.

Essential oil dilution is often a matter of "trial and error" but 1 drop of EO in 1 tablespoon of carrier oil (i.e. about 0.2% dilution) is typical for babies, infants and young children. In the case of adults, 2 drops of essential oil per teaspoon of carrier oil (0.75%) is more suitable although diluted mixtures may be better for individuals with sensitive skins. In massage therapy, dilutions of 2-5% are more common.

---

103   Fractionated coconut oil is coconut oil that has been treated to remove long-chain triglycerides to produce a thin, odorless, non-greasy liquid that is quickly absorbed by the skin; further, it does not interact with, or change the chemical composition of, the essential oil].

It should also be mentioned that it is not uncommon for certain companies to market what are claimed to be 100% pure natural essential oils. Unfortunately, many of these products have greater or lesser amounts of synthetic essential oils so that they are neither 100% pure nor are they natural. Based on anecdotal and apocryphal comments made to the author, these essential oils apparently often cause quite significant skin and other adverse effects and reactions. This subject will be returned to again below, but it appears that the incidence of adverse effects such as skin irritation is far lower with <u>100% pure natural</u> essential oils. Further, many of the most widely used essential oils for skin care, e.g. lavender oil and tea tree oil, have been used for literally thousands of years across the globe. It is inconceivable that such age-old practices would still be in regular and repeated use if adverse skin effects and dermatitis were common rather than the exception.

COSMETICS

Cosmetics, skin creams, shampoos and conditioners as well as lipsticks and lip-balms *may* contain irritant chemicals which are included in the misleading and all-encompassing designation of "fragrances". Many of these "fragrances" are synthetic products and can be hazardous, as mentioned in Chapter 13. Because of adverse skin reactions from cheap make-up imported from outside the U.S.A. (particularly some products manufactured for children!), many people might decide never to use any cosmetics again. While this may be an overreaction, even a partial listing of potentially hazardous chemicals in cosmetics and foods does indicate that educated and knowledgeable consumers can protect themselves by simply reading labels.

There are, in fact, many essential oils that are used in cosmetics, shampoos and conditioners to perform the same functions as the synthetic, cheaper and hazardous chemicals often used as "fragrances". These acceptable and probably beneficial additives include oil of rosemary, lavender oil, tea tree oil, jojoba oil, argan oil, aspen bark extract and grapefruit seed extract as well as honey. There are, of course, literally hundreds of other essential oils that have recognized and well-established benefits to the skin and hair, the mind and the body. These essential oils are common in massage therapy and aromatherapy, and are now increasingly being used in skin-care products, cosmetics and even in foods, as previously discussed.

It is interesting that most cosmetologists recommend selecting more expensive cosmetics because, in general, they contain a far lower percentage of potentially hazardous ingredients and a greater content of essential oils. In contrast, the purity and quality of lower-cost cosmetics, shampoos, etc. may be questionable. Further, when essential oils are used in "higher end" products, it is likely that they are 100% pure, natural products and that alone reduces the risk of adverse skin reactions. In other words, "high-end" products cost more because they are formulated with costlier but safer and hypoallergenic ingredients than their cheaper competition. In addition, high end products not only last longer, go further and are more effective, they generally do not contain synthetic essential oils which some cosmetologists claim can cause severe skin reactions.

ADVERSE SYSTEMIC REACTIONS

Hypersensitivity reactions to essential oils in organs other than the skin and respiratory tract (systemic allergic reactions) are rare and those that have been reported are poorly documented, and many such reactions are related to food "allergies", see Appendix G. Nevertheless, systemic allergic reactions to essential oils have been known in a very few cases.

The consensus of scientific and medical opinion is that adverse systemic reactions to essential oils are even rarer than dermatological reactions. However, as mentioned above, there are anecdotal remarks about how the products of one large essential oil producer caused itching, localized rashes (*urticaria*) and even migraine-type headaches from use of their products. This may be due to some of these products being synthetic rather than natural essential oils.

The widespread and very long-term use of essential oils in mouthwashes, e.g. eucalyptol, menthol, wintergreen (methyl salicylate) and thymol in Listerine®, certainly argues against systemic effects from essential oils being commonplace. Further, numerous essential oils are certified as GRAS (Generally Recognized as Safe) by the FDA for oral consumption, Table 16.3.

Angelica	Eucalyptus globulus	Pepper
Basil	Idaho Blue Spruce	Peppermint
Bergamot	Juniper	Petitgrain
Chamomile, Roman	Jasmine	Pine
Chamomile, German	Laurus nobilis	Rosemary
Cinnamon Bark	Lavender	Rose
Citrus rind (all)	Lemon	Savory
Clary Sage	Lemongrass	Sage
Clove	Lime	Sandalwood
Coriander	Melissa (lemon balm)	Spearmint
Dill	Marjoram	Spruce
Frankincense	Myrrh	Tarragon
Galbanum	Myrtle	Tangerine
Geranium	Nutmeg	Thyme
Ginger	Orange	Valerian
Grapefruit	Oregano	Vetiver
Hyssop	Patchouli	Ylang Ylang

Table 16.3 Essential oils certified as Generally Recognized as Safe (GRAS) by the FDA for oral consumption

One interesting and rather debatable adverse systemic reaction to essential oils surfaced in an article, entitled "*More evidence essential oils make male breasts develop*", published in the New Scientist[104] in March 2018. This article referred to two published scientific papers that suggested some cases of male gynecomastia (abnormal breast growth) coincided with topical exposure to the oils. Apparently, this reaction occurred because the two essential oils (lavender and tea tree oil) boost estrogen (the female hormone) and inhibit testosterone (the male hormone).

One study, back in 2007, reported a suspected link between abnormal breast growth (*gynecomastia*) in 3 young boys and topical exposure to lavender and tea tree oils. In one case, a 4-year old boy had been experiencing symptoms for 2-3 weeks after his mother had

---

104   New Scientist is a weekly, London-based news magazine that covers all aspects of science and technology.

recently begun applying a lavender oil-containing "healing balm" to his skin. In a second case, a 10-year old boy had been developing enlarged breast tissue over the previous five months from using a shampoo and hair gel containing lavender oil and tea tree oil every morning. A 3rd boy, aged seven, had a one-month history of gynecomastia, ascribed to using lavender-scented soaps and skin lotions whereas his twin who had used the soap, but not the lotions, and had not developed the condition. When each of the boys stopped using the suspect products, the abnormal tissue growth subsided.

Interestingly, a second study, published in 2016, also reported gynecomastia in 3 pre-pubescent boys. Apparently, the cause was suspected to be the use of a lavender oil-containing cologne that is popular with Hispanic communities within the U.S.A. It was noted, however, that laboratory-based tests on rats did not produce this effect. Medical evaluation of the affected children, however, showed no change in the levels of the usual hormones circulating in their bodies.

Gynecomastia is rare, and there is often no obvious cause although the consensus opinion is that it is related to a hormone imbalance. In fact, it is well-established that hormone levels in pre-pubescent males are particularly sensitive to changes. Whether essential oils within soaps and hair-care products can cause gynecomastia would appear to be a significant "stretch". Even though essential oils have been used in cosmetics for thousands of years, no comparable systemic effects have ever been reported anecdotally or otherwise, and no recognized authority on essential oils has ever subscribed to the notion that essential oils have any effect on puberty. In fact, there is a growing body of evidence that environmental effects and a wide variety of food additives and questionable chemicals present in foodstuffs are strongly influencing children approaching or going through puberty.

In conclusion, it is possible that topical exposure to, and ingestion of, essential oils *may* cause dermatological or systemic effects, but such instances appear to be very rare. Further, any such effects appear to resolve without incident when exposure is reduced or stopped.

CHAPTER 17

PREBIOTICS, PROBIOTICS and GASTRIC HEALTH

A basic tenet of the 21st Century is that sound mental and physical health requires a balanced and nutritious diet, regular exercise, a stress-free environment and strong interpersonal relationships. The reality for most people, however, is much different and diabetes, coronary artery disease, obesity and many other life-threatening conditions are rampant. Modern man has been abusing the digestive system for decades, and the situation is becoming steadily worse. Dietary factors, i.e. the food we eat and the beverages we drink, directly and usually adversely impact gut health, with the many stresses of the modern world only compounding the problems.

It is not surprising, therefore, that we are inundated with a constant barrage of advertisements on the Internet and in all the media regarding the benefits of vitamins, minerals, "superfoods" and, latterly, probiotics. Although the virtues of these dietary factors are extolled daily, it is not altogether clear just how they work or what they do for us.

Gastric health is important, as most sufferers from constipation, diarrhea, indigestion, acid reflux, heart burn or simple stomach aches will testify. Not only that, most of us are aware of the old adage that "an apple a day keeps the doctor away" although quite why that may be the case is unclear. As always, the situation regarding internal or systemic health is rather more complex than that when it comes to the gastrointestinal (G.I.) tract, commonly referred to as the digestive system, our intestines and the gut.

In fact, at least 75-80% and probably a higher percentage of the body's immune system originates in the gut, so intestinal health and vitality is very important for the body's wellbeing and overall health. This is where diet, essential oils, prebiotics and probiotics come into play. Consequently, it might be useful to provide a brief introduction to the gastro-intestinal (GI) tract and how it works. It should be noted that whereas the "gut" is technically the intestines, the term is now commonly used interchangeably to designate the entire digestive system.

THE G.I. SYSTEM

The alimentary system or the digestive tract is basically one long tube that traverses the entire body, shown schematically in Figure 17.1. It starts at the mouth and ends at the anus with the pharynx, esophagus, stomach, ileum (small intestine), colon (large intestine) and the rectum between the two ends.

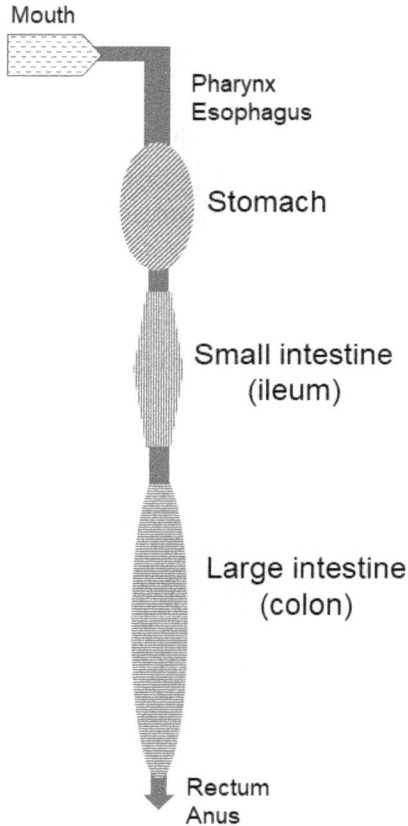

Figure 17.1 Schematic diagram of the human digestive system.

The entry portal to the digestive system is the oral cavity or mouth. Various glands supply the mouth with saliva, exuding about 1.5 to 2 liters per day. Saliva contains certain proteins and enzymes; the latter are substances produced by the body which act as catalysts to bring about specific biochemical reactions. The enzymes supplied by saliva initiate the digestive processes during mastication (chewing). Saliva also performs other essential functions, notably helping rinse foodstuffs from the teeth, maintaining the oral pH or acidity close to neutrality to reduce acid attack on the teeth, and helping remineralize the teeth to offset damage caused by acidic attack. The oral cavity also contains high concentrations of multiple species of micro-organisms, many of which are beneficial whereas others are potentially harmful. The concentration and variety of these bacterial species will vary with the individual depending upon diet, oral hygiene and the presence of dental prostheses (e.g. bridges and dentures).

After mastication, food and liquids are passed through the esophagus into the stomach where ingested food and liquids are collected. After interacting with stomach acids and various enzymes, the partially digested material, a thick, semifluid mass known as *chyme*, is passed in small amounts into the small intestine, also known as the small bowel.

The small intestine is a tightly folded tube about 20 ft (6 m) in length that is connected to the stomach at the top end and the large intestine (colon) at the lower end. The entire length of the small intestine is wrapped by smooth muscle which helps transport food through the bowel by a pulsing process known as *peristalsis*. The inner surfaces of the small intestine have numerous folds covered in projecting filaments (*villi*) which greatly increase the surface area and facilitate absorption of nutrients from the gut. In contrast to the acidic (low pH) conditions of the stomach, the pH in the small intestine is usually between 7 and 8, i.e., neutral to weakly alkaline. The schematic diagram of the digestive system in Figure 17.1 shows the alimentary (digestive) system as a straight connection between mouth and anus but within the body, the large intestine follows a quasi-rectangular path that surrounds the small intestine.

The bulk of the food that passes from the stomach is digested and absorbed in the small intestine and the extracted nutrients include fructose, amino acids, small peptides, carbohydrates, vitamins, most glucose molecules and fats. The overall digestion process results in individual food components being absorbed into the blood stream and carried throughout the body.

Residues from the small bowel are then moved by muscle contraction (peristalsis) into the large bowel (the large intestine or colon), a structure approximately 5 feet (1.5 meter) in length. Ultimately, the residue is moved to the rectum and evacuated. Until comparatively recently, the colon commonly was regarded as a waste depository for food residues despite being extensively colonized by bacteria. It is now recognized that the colonic microorganisms (the flora or microorganisms present within the colon) are essential components in the re-absorption of water that occurs within the colon. So, in fact, the colon is far more than just a dumping ground for food residues.

MICROFLORA OF THE GI TRACT

As already stated, some 75-80% of the cells of the immune system reside within the small and large intestines. Under normal circumstances, the gastrointestinal tract contains a balanced number of beneficial ("good") and potentially harmful ("bad") bacteria. This collection of micro-organisms is known as the normal (or natural) microflora or microbiome and, in the healthy individual, there is a balance between good and bad bacteria. Any imbalance between the good and bad bacteria is known as *dysbiosis*[105], and such imbalances cause gastric problems which can impair the immune system.

The small and large intestines contain multiple species of Gram-positive and Gram-negative rods and cocci (see Appendix F). These bacteria assist the absorption of nutrients, facilitate absorption of calcium and magnesium and generate short-chain fatty acids which help regenerate the colon wall. Further, the "good" bacteria also help make vitamin K and maintain proper functioning of the immune system. Not only that, these good bacteria help prevent hypersensitivity reactions such as allergies and asthma as well as reduce triglyceride levels within the blood.

In general, micro-organisms in the proximal (right) side of the colon, known as the ascending colon, grow at a fast rate because of a good supply of nutrients. The bacterial fermentation products of digested nutrients, the short chain fatty acids mentioned above, lower the pH, i.e. increase the acidity, in the colon. In contrast, bacteria in the distal (left) side of the colon (known as the descending colon) have a more restricted nutrient supply and grow more slowly so that the pH approaches neutrality. It should be mentioned, in passing, that the stomach was previously considered to be sterile due to its acidity. It is now recognized that certain bacteria such as the pathogenic *Helicobacter*

---

105   *Dysbiosis:* scientific/medical term for a microbial imbalance (or maladaptation) on or inside the body; a common example of dysbiosis is an impaired microbiota such as the community of microorganisms in the G.I. tract.

pylori (*H. pylori*) can be found in large numbers in the stomach of some individuals and, in fact, *H. pylori* infects the stomachs of roughly 60% of the world's adult population. While *H. pylori* infections are usually harmless, they do tend to attack the stomach lining and are responsible for most ulcers in the stomach and small intestine.

Some of the bacterial species populating the colon may cause disease under certain circumstances. These potential pathogens ("bad" bacteria) actively compete with beneficial bacteria in colonizing the colon and the relative concentrations of beneficial *vs.* pathogenic bacteria can impact health. An example of this is the toxin-producing microorganism, *Clostridium difficile*. When present at low levels, *C. difficile* causes minimal if any side-effects but when present at high concentrations, it can cause life-threatening disease. Other less desirable bacteria also present in the gut convert sulfur-containing compounds in foods to hydrogen sulfide (H_2S), a poisonous gas with an offensive smell. In fact, the rotten egg smell of flatus (the gas we emit sometime after eating) is due to hydrogen sulfide and has been related to the prevalence of ulcerative colitis.

DIGESTIVE AND GASTRIC ISSUES

Although the heathy gut has a proper balance in the numbers and types of intestinal bacteria, several factors can upset this delicate balance, including poor diet, natural aging, stress and antibiotic therapy. A preponderance of "bad" bacteria can be caused, for example, by elevated intestinal pH, i.e. a more alkaline environment and this is why taking antacids for "indigestion" may alleviate symptoms for a short time but does not "cure" the condition. Further, if a bacterial imbalance leads to an overgrowth or preponderance of bad bacteria and yeast within the gut, *intestinal dyspepsia*[106] can set in.

Dysbiosis may also result in Small Intestine Bacterial Overgrowth (SIBO) which occurs when colonic bacteria are found in the small intestine. It is now recognized that dysbiosis and, particularly, SIBO

---

106 *Dyspepsia*: A condition having various upper abdominal symptoms including pain, bloating, feeling unusually full after meals even with little intake of food, loss of appetite, heartburn, regurgitation of food or acid, and nausea. *Dyspepsia* often is caused by a stomach ulcer or acid reflux disease.

are connected with other health concerns, including IBS (irritable bowel syndrome) and metabolic disorders.

At one time, irritable bowel syndrome (IBS) was a blanket term applied by physicians to gastric conditions with no apparent cause despite the fact that it affects more than 10% of the global population. Interestingly, some 30% of IBS sufferers never actually seek a proper diagnosis of their condition. Although IBS is usually managed with diet and medication, essential oils have been indicated for symptom control, as discussed below.

Heartburn, also known as acid indigestion, is the most common symptom of acid reflux or GERD[107]. Sufferers usually experience a burning chest pain that starts behind the breastbone ("heartburn") and then moves upward to the neck and throat, and some people may also experience an acidic or bitter taste and sometimes a burning sensation in the mouth or throat. GERD has two causes, namely a faulty "flap" that allows gastric acids to back-up into the esophagus and/or there might be too much or a decreased amount of stomach acids. The latter can be affected by lifestyle and diet, as well as bacteria.

Finally, a common gastric problem is nausea, the symptoms of which can range from being simply unpleasant to have a debilitating effect. Nausea is often associated with several ailments and conditions including poor diet, dysbiosis as well as lifestyle issues.

ESSENTIAL OILS FOR GASTRIC PROBLEMS

The tendency for gastric health sufferers to opt for natural remedies, notably essential oils, to alleviate problems parallels trends in other areas of medicine. Many gastric-related claims are made for enteric-coated peppermint oil as well as oregano, ginger and fennel capsules, notably that they support a healthy digestion, promote a better balance of intestinal flora, soothe stomach upsets as well as reduce gas emissions. However, at this time, there is insufficient data to substantiate

---

107 *GERD* (gastro-esophageal reflux disease) arises when the esophageal sphincter (a circular muscle that constricts a natural body passage or orifice, but which relaxes as required by normal physiological functioning) loosens abnormally or weakens. This allows stomach acid to flow back up into the esophagus, causing "heartburn".

these claims or to recommend them as a standard treatment for any condition. What is known regarding essential oils and gastric health is briefly reviewed here but the basic rule should be to consult a health-care provider before embarking on self-medication, particularly with children or during pregnancy.

The scientific literature indicates that certain essential oils can have beneficial effects on gut dysbiosis, i.e. intestinal bacterial imbalance, because they can curb the proliferation of pathogenic bacteria while having no adverse effects on beneficial bacteria. The essential oils reported to be notably advantageous include peppermint, caraway, ginger, bitter orange and lavender. The important point is that using essential oils to alleviate nausea and the symptoms of GERD, IBS, SIBO and other intestinal flora issues <u>may</u> provide relief of symptoms without damaging the "good" bacteria in the gut.

Clinical studies indicate that peppermint oil, together with dietary fiber, has the same efficacy in treating IBS as the antispasmodic medications commonly prescribed for this purpose. This effectiveness is particularly true for enteric-coated peppermint capsules, the enteric coating permitting the capsules to pass through the stomach without damage by gastric acids Overall, the evidence suggests that peppermint oil is generally safe when used appropriately but it can cause stomach upsets and even a burning sensation in the rectum. High doses are thought to cause nausea, heart problems, loss of appetite and nervous system issues, with large amounts of peppermint oil being potentially toxic, leading to renal failure and death. At this time, the optimal levels of peppermint supplements are not known.

Peppermint oil supplements are contraindicated when pregnant or breastfeeding and should not be used if potential users have liver disease, inflammation of the gallbladder, gallstones or obstruction of the bile ducts. Further, peppermint oil supplements should not be used by sufferers from ulcers, chronic heartburn or hiatal hernia. Peppermint oil should <u>not</u> be used by GERD sufferers because it can relax the muscles of the esophagus, one cause of the condition. This effect on the esophageal muscles would only exacerbate the problem.

Studies indicate that one approach to dealing with GERD is through essential oils that protect the stomach lining and improve digestive processes. It appears that ginger, in concert with turmeric, reduces damage done to the stomach wall and can increase antioxidant levels. The beneficial action of ginger on gut health has been recognized for centuries by Japanese chefs who regularly accompany sushi and other dishes with ginger as a boost to the digestive system.

Sufferers from nausea can experience numerous symptoms, ranging in intensity from unpleasant to debilitating. Worse, the prevalence of nausea appears to be increasing, possibly because of poor diet as well as the effects of modern lifestyles. As most nausea sufferers are aware, scent can have a major effect in either a positive or negative way on how they feel. Consequently, inhaled essential oils can be an effective approach to managing nausea almost regardless of the specific cause. In particular, peppermint and ginger work well together in alleviating nausea, as do citrus oils such as bitter orange. Studies show that inhaling lemon is highly effective in alleviating morning sickness/nausea during pregnancy. Diffusers, nasal inhalers as well as aroma sticks (rattan diffuser reeds immersed in essential oils) are all good approaches to nausea relief.

Finally, recent research indicates that there is increasing evidence that certain essential oils can create a synergistic effect[108] when coupled with probiotics. As a result of this interaction, there appear to be increased benefits compared to either the essential oil or probiotic alone. Research studies are continuing in this area.

PROBIOTICS

It is interesting that only a few years ago, virtually no-one had even heard of probiotics but now they seem to be everywhere. Big Pharma and numerous smaller pharmaceutical companies market probiotics, and even pet foods now contain them. Commercials and advertisements extolling the health benefits of probiotics appear daily on television and in virtually every magazine and newspaper. Nevertheless, information on these bacterial workhorses is generally limited for the general public and even less information is available on prebiotics, the agents that can increase the numbers of probiotics in the gut. Although

---

108 *Synergistic effect*: the term applied when there is an interaction or cooperation between two or more agents to produce a combined effect greater than the sum of their separate effects.

the latter are discussed below, the combined effect of these dietary components can have a major and often beneficial impact on the human gut and overall (systemic) health.

Probiotics[109,110] are microorganisms that reside in the intestines and which have no parasitic effect on man. These *enteric* microorganisms are of vital importance to health but for probiotics to be truly effective, the diet must also contain prebiotics, as discussed later.

Western interest in probiotics stems from the pioneering work in Bulgaria of a Russian physician, Eli Metchnikoff, during the early years of the 20th Century. Metchnikoff showed a relationship between the exceptional vitality and unusually long lives of Bulgarian people and their consumption of large amounts of natural yoghurt. He was able to identify certain microorganisms (later termed *probiotics*) which were present in yoghurt. Metchnikoff's findings were supported by the long-held tradition of physicians in the Near- and Middle East to treat digestive (gastrointestinal) disorders, liver problems and poor appetite with soured milk, a precursor of yoghurt. In fact, soured milk, yoghurt and many native fermented beverages have been an integral part of the daily diet in parts of Europe and the Middle East for centuries.

Consuming probiotic foods benefits the gut because they inhibit the growth of pathogenic microorganisms, i.e. "bad" bacteria. Basically, anything that protects the body and, notably, the gut against pathogenic bacteria will provide a positive stimulus to the immune system. Another important aspect of consuming probiotics is that when combined with indigestible carbohydrates known as prebiotics (see below), there is a dramatic effect on constipation as well as many other gastric conditions.

Since the groundbreaking work of Metchnikoff, many other probiotic functional foods have been identified and it is now widely accepted that certain microorganisms, notably those derived from fer-

---

109 Probiotics are defined by the World Health Organization (WHO) and the Food and Agricultural Organization of the United Nations (FAO) as living microorganisms which confer health benefits on the host when administered in adequate amounts. Now, they are accepted to be concentrated supplements of live microbial foods that benefit the host.

110 J. A. von Fraunhofer: Prebiotics and Probiotics. CreateSpace, Seattle, WA (2012).

mented milk products, are beneficial to both the health and viability of
the GI tract and the whole body. These include a lactic acid-fermented
oatmeal gruel consumed in Sweden, the Tanzanian beverage, Togwa,
and the fermented milk drink, Kefir. The latter has been consumed for
hundreds of years in the Caucasus region because of the strongly-held
belief that it helps maintain the strength of the stomach and immune
system although the immune system obviously was unheard of when
Kefir was first produced and consumed on a regular basis.

PREBIOTICS

Most people are unfamiliar with the term prebiotics although they are
simply high fiber foodstuffs which are not digested by the enzymes and
acids in the stomach and pass virtually intact into the colon. Because
of this, they have minimal caloric value, i.e. have no nutritional effect,
and do not increase serum glucose or stimulate insulin secretion.
However, once the prebiotic fibers enter the colon, they are digested by
the colonic microflora, producing short chain fatty acids., which feed
probiotic bacteria.

One of the first to explore the beneficial effects of starch-free fruits
and green leafy vegetables was Arnold Ehret[111] who claimed that a diet
of raw fruits and green-leaf vegetables are "non-mucus" producers. He
suggested that these foodstuffs together with a regimen of long- and
short-term fasting results in effective colonic irrigation. This regimen
was based on his finding that a vegetarian diet cured his Bright's disease (a kidney disease), a condition deemed incurable by the numerous
eminent physicians that he consulted. Ehret then went on to explore
natural healing and holistic medicine, advocating vegetarianism as a
method of cleansing and repairing the body when afflicted by poor
nutrition and over-eating. The importance of "colonic irrigation" was
emphasized when Ehret, and fellow physician Bernard Jensen, performed numerous autopsies and found that 90 - 95% of autopsied
patients had clogged colons and most had suffered from chronic constipation during their lives. This pioneering work of Ehret, and the

---

111 Arnold Ehret (1866–1922) is considered to be the "father" of naturopathic
medicine and wrote a ground-breaking book entitled the *Mucusless Diet Healing
System.*

findings of subsequent researchers, led to studies directed at the effect of fibrous foods on health.

The concept of *prebiotics* was first introduced by Gibson and Roberfroid[112]. They published their work, "Dietary modulation of the human colonic microbiota: introducing the concept of prebiotics", in the Journal of Nutrition in 1995 and it was a landmark contribution to the science of nutrition.

Although prebiotics were originally described as non-digestible functional foods that stimulated the growth or activity of bacteria in the digestive system, they are now defined as "a selectively fermented dietary ingredient". This selective fermentation allows specific changes in both the composition and activity of the gastrointestinal microflora, conferring benefits upon the health of the host.

Typically, prebiotics are carbohydrates and the most important of these are known as fructooligosaccharides (FOS), namely oligofructose[113] and inulin. Although other functional foodstuffs may be described as "prebiotic", these are more commonly referred to as "possible prebiotics", "likely prebiotics" or "having prebiotic activity". While many dietary fibers such as digestion-resistant starch and non-starch polysaccharides provide substrates for fermentation by colonic bacteria, only fructooligosaccharides truly meet the criteria to qualify as prebiotics.

So, prebiotics are soluble fibers and common dietary sources of prebiotic fibers, are indicated in Table 17.1.

---

112 G. R. Gibson and M. B. Roberfroid worked at the Medical Research Council Dunn Nutrition Centre in Cambridge, England.

113 *Oligofructose* is a dietary fiber found in vegetables and other plants that is a subgroup of inulin. Oligofructose, better known as a fructooligosaccharide (FOS), is often used as a sweetener with sweetness levels of 30-50% of sugar but minimal calories. Inulin is a natural blend of fructose (sugar) polymers found widely distributed in nature as plant storage carbohydrates.

Agave	Jerusalem artichoke
Asparagus	Leeks
Bananas	Oats
Barley	Onions
Belgian endive root	Soybeans
Chicory root	Wheat
Garlic	Wild yam

Table 17.1 Common sources of inulin and dietary prebiotics.

Interestingly, over 200 oligosaccharides[114] occur naturally in human breast milk and contribute to the immune system of the breast-fed baby. Several leading organism-engineering and biotech firms are now developing "human milk oligosaccharides" (HMOs) for use in infant formula and other foods. Early research findings indicate that these HMOs are effective in the treatment of Crohn's disease, irritable bowel syndrome and damage to the gut microbiota caused by antibiotics.

PROBIOTIC SPECIES

Since the early 20th Century, a great many probiotic bacterial species have been identified and each species or genus can comprise up to hundreds of separate strains[115]. The genus, *Lactobacillus*, for example, comprises at least 60 species and is the fermentation agent used for flavoring and as a preservative in foods like sauerkraut and sausage.

---

114 An *oligosaccharide* is a saccharide polymer containing a small number (typically 3 to 10) of monosaccharides or simple sugars. *Oligosaccharides* can have many biological functions including cell recognition and cell binding. Note that the word saccharide is a synonym for carbohydrate and used for either simple sugars or polymers such as starch and cellulose.

115 *Genus* is the scientific term for a group of closely-related species, that is, the largest group of organisms that can interbreed to produce a fertile offspring. A *strain* is a genetic variant or subtype of a micro-organism (e.g., a bacterium or virus) and, for example, a "flu *strain*" is a certain *biological* form or variant of the influenza virus.

Each probiotic bacterial strain may have different characteristics and, consequently, their health benefit effects can vary markedly. Many species, notably those of the genus *Lactobacillus,* are common in the mucosa that extends from the mouth to the anus in humans. Many naturally-occurring bacteria in the gut promote healthy GI microbial systems by producing lactic acid which helps digest foods, improves the bioavailability of minerals and supports production of B vitamins within the body. This is important for lactose-intolerant individuals because the bacteria produce enzymes which break down lactose, clearly benefiting the digestive health of the individual.

Many probiotic formulations are available from pharmacies, health food stores and internet sites and, increasingly, major food manufacturers market yoghurts that contain these "protective" or health-conferring bacteria. Although probiotic formulations and their bacterial counts may differ with the manufacturer, most products contain one or more of the most commonly used probiotics, indicated in Table 17.2. Commercial probiotic formulations generally contain several different species so that while one particular strain might not work for a given individual, others present in the formulation should be effective.

Lactobacillus acidophilus
Lactobacillus bifidum
Lactobacillus brevis
Lactobacillus bulgaricus
Lactobacillus casei
Lactobacillus gasseri
Lactobacillus helveticus
Lactobacillus infantis
Lactobacillus lactis
Lactobacillus longum
Lactobacillus paracasei
Lactobacillus plantarum
Lactobacillus rhamnosus
Lactobacillus salivarius
Bacillus coagluans

Bifidobacterium bifidum   *Bifidobacterium breve*   *Bifidobacterium lactis*   *Bifidobacterium longum*   *Bifidus regularis*
Pediococcus acidilactici
Saccharomyces boulandii
Streptococcus salivarius   *Streptococcus thermophilus*

Table 17.2 Widely used probiotic bacteria

PROBIOTICS AND GI HEALTH

The normal, indigenous microflora in healthy people limits invasion and overgrowth by pathogenic bacteria. The intrinsic stability or equilibrium between "good" and "bad" bacterial species in the gut, however, can be disrupted by many factors, notably poor nutrition (i.e. an unbalanced diet) and the ingestion of antibiotics, antacids and alcohol. Psychological stress also affects bacterial balance within the digestive system and one consequence of the increasing pressures experienced in the 21st Century is that gastric ulcers, and their associated bacteria (*H. pylori*), are now relatively common afflictions.

Any significant reduction in the numbers of individual components of the bacterial population in the gut can result in overgrowth by previously suppressed minority elements. The common symptoms associated with such overgrowth are bloating, abdominal pain, increased flatulence and diarrhea.

Interestingly, a complication of the increasingly common gastric bypass surgery treatment for obesity can be an alteration in the gastrointestinal flora which may lead to bacterial overgrowth. It was found, however, that probiotic supplementation following gastric bypass surgery prevented bacterial overgrowth, and patients had a greater weight loss and a 50% higher level of vitamin B-12 than those not taking probiotics. In this vein, a study was conducted in France on women suffering from regular digestive problems rather than gastrointestinal diseases. One group received yogurt supplemented with probiotics and the other a non-fermented dairy product. After a month, improvements in gastrointestinal health (digestive symptoms and comfort) was found for women receiving the probiotic yogurt but the benefits from probiotics disappeared within a month after cessation of supplementation. This suggests that continued probiotics supplementation is necessary to maintain gastrointestinal well-being.

Several studies indicate that probiotics can help prevent and treat diarrhea, even for patients on antibiotics. Antibiotic-related diarrhea is relatively common (i.e. a prevalence of 20-30%) with children, and many parents stop antibiotic therapy for their children or seek further medical treatment to alleviate the diarrhea. There is evidence, however, that the antibiotic-rich kefir can treat or prevent antibiotic-induced diarrhea, and appears to be very effective with younger, sicker children. This may be the result of boosting the immune system, which may be less necessary for healthier pediatric patients. There are also indications that the duration of episodes of acute watery diarrhea in children caused by the rotavirus is decreased by several types of probiotics.

These beneficial effects of probiotics may be due to their ability to recolonize the intestinal microflora which protects the stomach lining. This in turn reduces the severity of acute diarrhea in children as well as preventing/treating antibiotic-associated diarrhea and inflammatory bowel disease. *Lactobacillus salivarius*, for example, may be a potentially effective probiotic against *Helicobacter pylori (H. pylori)*, a bacterium that causes chronic low-level inflammation, ulcers and stomach cancer. However, other scientific work suggests that because probiotic bacteria *per se* may not be able to eliminate *H. pylori,* other effects may be operating.

Although most scientific probiotics studies have focused on the prevention and treatment of gastrointestinal disease and allergies, there is a growing number of claims that probiotics are effective against other conditions, Table 17.3.

Alleviation of digestive disorders
Control of pathogenic bacteria
Control of yeasts
Diminished gas, bloating and abdominal pain
Diminished irritable bowel syndrome
Enhanced metabolization of B vitamins
Immune system enhancement
Improve immune function
Improved absorption of calcium and magnesium
Improved digestion
Prevention and treatment of diarrhea
Prevention and treatment of pediatric respiratory infections
Prevention of recurrence of superficial bladder cancer
Relief of constipation and diarrhea
Reduction in some allergic reactions
Restoration of natural microflora balance after stress,
antibiotic therapy, alcohol use and chemotherapy.

Table 17.3 Common health benefit claims of probiotics therapy

In other words, the health effects of ingested probiotic micro-organisms are not confined to the intestinal tract because many systemic health problems originate, at least in part, from adverse conditions within the colon and their effect on the immune system. These problems include yeast-associated conditions, ulcers, dermatitis, acne, sinus problems, allergies, halitosis, colds, influenza and other problems involving the immune system. Headaches and anxiety/mood swings also have been ascribed to bacterial imbalance within the colon.

The wider health benefit claims in Table 17.3 are based on the presumption that by maintaining or improving the barrier function of the intestinal mucosa, probiotics may inhibit translocation of potential pathogens. This should prevent infections of the blood stream and the correlated adverse effects on other tissues and organs. However, as mentioned elsewhere, changes in microbial balance arising from exogenous bacteria may be transient and of limited effectiveness. The effectiveness of probiotics in controlling yeast infections, for example, is debatable.

Supporting data for the claims that probiotics can alleviate and possibly cure the conditions indicated in Table 17.3 are not always clear-cut or scientifically validated. On the other hand, because some 80% of the body's immune cells are located within the gut and probiotics may ensure a healthy balance of the intestinal microflora, there is a logical basis for claims regarding their beneficial effects upon the immune system. Further, because probiotics appear to have an anti-inflammatory action, they may be helpful for patients suffering from various types of inflammatory or autoimmune diseases.

In the overall context of probiotics and health, it must be borne in mind that probiotics and other supplements commonly are consumed by healthy and health-conscious people. However, it is somewhat ironic that little is known about the effect of probiotics on the immune system of the healthy individual.

It should also be noted that probiotics are living organisms and, consequently, manufacturers must adhere to certain guidelines. These include careful storage and packaging to protect them from light, air, elevated temperatures and moisture. Also, probiotic supplements must contain very large numbers of living microorganisms so that there must be enough left after transiting the acids and digestive enzymes in the stomach and small intestine to survive and still be viable once they reach the colon. Consequently, enteric coatings and specialized encapsulation techniques are used with probiotic supplements to help preserve the viability of probiotic bacteria on passage through the stomach and small intestine to the colon. It should be noted that the use of antacids should be avoided because they raise the intestinal pH, which tends to kill the bacteria.

The optimal number of bacteria to be taken daily is unknown but it appears that *more is better than less* to compensate for destruction of the ingested bacteria on transit through the stomach and intestines, as noted above. Because it is not known which strains of probiotic bacteria are the most effective, most manufacturers formulate supplements containing up to 10-15 different strains to satisfy individual needs. Also, current thinking is that probiotics capsules must contain at least 5 billion (5×10^9) cfu (colony-forming units) to be effective.

Finally, when prebiotics and probiotics are combined, they are known as *synbiotics* because they work together. Supplement bottle labelling will indicate that inulin or a fructooligosaccharide is present in the supplement capsules. Interestingly, there is increasing evidence that not only that probiotics may rely upon prebiotics to achieve maximal effectiveness, but that it appears that prebiotics alone are effective in stimulating the immune system. In other words, parental admonitions for their children to eat vegetables and the old adage regarding apples and doctors now are reinforced by science and hark back to the resurrected teachings of Ehret and the health benefits of vegetarianism.

CHAPTER 18

PACKAGING and SHIPPING

Young Living produces a very large number of individual essential oils (referred to as "singles" in their Product Guide) together with many different oil blends as well as a wide variety of products that are based on, or contain, essential oils. The latter include, but are not limited to, products that support wellness, comfort the spirit, beautify the skin and hair, wash the face and body, nourish the skin, and clean the home. Company products may be purchased from some retail stores but, predominantly, they are available from Young Living members. Given the multiplicity of Young Living products, the over six (6) million global membership and a growing number of International Offices, it is no surprise that Young Living is an universally-known, highly respected household name and a leading company in the essential oil industry.

ORGANIZATION

To satisfy the ever-increasing demands of the world-wide market, an incredible organization exists to produce, test, package and ship Young Living products. There are many interactive structures and components within that organization, Figure 18.1. The primary component is obviously production which includes the many subjects discussed in this book. However, what is manufactured, namely individual essential

oils, essential oil blends and the numerous other Young Living products as well as the quantities of each category of items produced every
year, is determined by what are loosely termed Marketing and Sales in
Figure 18.1.

Marketing, at least in part, generates the demand for new and
existing products and these are available to members through Sales.

MARKETING

Marketing encompasses pricing, public relations (PR), promotions,
informational flyers, graphics and advertising. Input from members
and Young Living staff as well as external consultants and technical
experts collectively provide inspiration for new and innovative products. The latter are introduced each year at the frequently held retreats
and conventions. The interactions and interdependence of Production,
Marketing and Sales as well as Young Living members are vital to the
Company and its success.

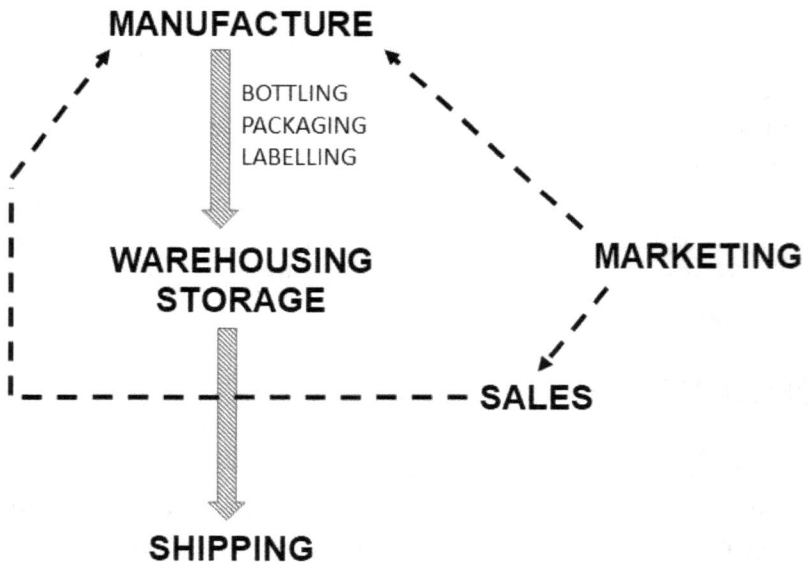

Figure 18.1 Schematic of the Organization of Young Living

SALES

Member retreats and National and International conventions constitute part of the remit of Sales. Feedback from members is of major importance to Marketing and Production, and has a bearing on the Sales, Warehousing, and Shipping operations. *Sales* is a somewhat loose description of the part of the organization that includes receiving and dispatching orders, providing product advice to members as well as answering questions on a variety of issues. *Sales* also provides technical and marketing support for the millions of Young Living members throughout the world.

Central to successful sales of products for any company is the availability, quality and price of the goods offered for sale, with price often being a large factor in the selection of any purchase by consumers. Establishing the price of any item for sale involves many different factors, summarized in Figure 18.2. In the case of essential oils, the cost of raw materials, notably the planting, growing and harvesting of crops as well as extracting the oils from their botanical sources and the cost of utilities and transportation are major components of pricing calculations.

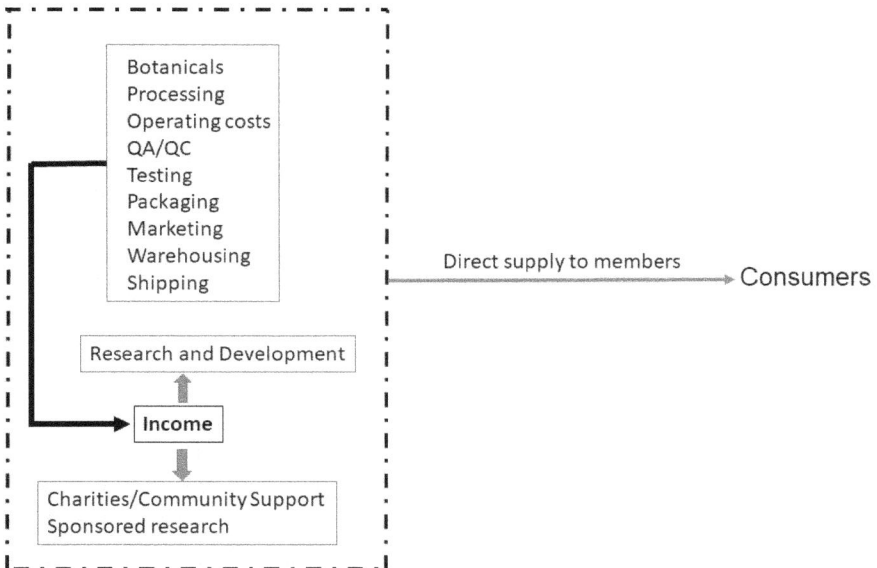

Figure 18.2 Basic economics of production, marketing and pricing of products.

A major advantage with Young Living and its huge network of members is that there is no wholesale distributor between Young Living and its members. This approach eliminates the additional overhead, profit and taxes added to the base price from other essential oil producers and ensures that Young Living can achieve the lowest possible product cost and greatest value for its members. Further, by eliminating the intermediary middleman, members can order items directly from Young Living which are shipped to them from Warehousing, ensuring prompt and timely delivery.

Another important consideration with the way Young Living and its membership is structured is how that "profit" earned from Sales is used. Not only are significant sums donated to charity each year, but there is little need to set aside revenue to service debt and, consequently, part of the profit is ploughed back into the Company. This is used to finance Research and Development as well as Young Living's support for National and International charities, disaster relief efforts and community involvement. Further, Young Living can provide sponsorship for many research organizations that rely upon corporate donations and support to advance scientific research and build knowledge.

It should also be apparent from Figure 18.2 and the many comments made throughout this book that a considerable amount of effort, energy, capital expenditure and operating costs are involved in producing essential oils. Consequently, the discerning reader and user of Young Living essential oils will wonder how retailers can market bottles of "essential oils" for just a few dollars and expect them to be pure and natural.

PACKAGING

Critical to the essential oil industry are the bottling and packaging operations. The bottling process involves various sizes of bottles and containers which are used to contain multiple individual essential oils and oil blends as well as a variety of other liquids such as shower gels, liquid soaps, hair care products and the tonic, Ningxia. Young Living also produces a large array of creams and pastes that must be injected into different sizes of containers. Further, many products are shipped in tubs, small jars and tubes. In other words, the operation and maintenance of numerous filling equipment stations for many different liquids and pastes is a very large-scale and demanding process.

In the case of liquids to be shipped in glass containers, the bottles must be cleaned, sanitized, dried and blasted free of any residue and debris using compressed air before any bottling can be undertaken. Then they are fed to the filling station before being delivered to the capping and labelling station.

Depending on the magnitude of the bottling process, i.e., the number of bottles to be filled as well as the volume of oil or other liquid product injected into each bottle, different types of bottling machinery are used. Liquid level machines inject the oil into the bottles so that they are filled to the same level with every bottle whereas volumetric filling machines fill each bottle with the same amount of liquid. Depending on the numbers of bottles involved and the volumes of oil being bottled, the bottles can be filled with pressure hoses or gravity-fed machines. Since the bottling process is automated, inline filling machines are most popular whereas rotary bottle-feed machines are much faster but more expensive to set up. After filling, the bottles are then passed to the capping and labelling station.

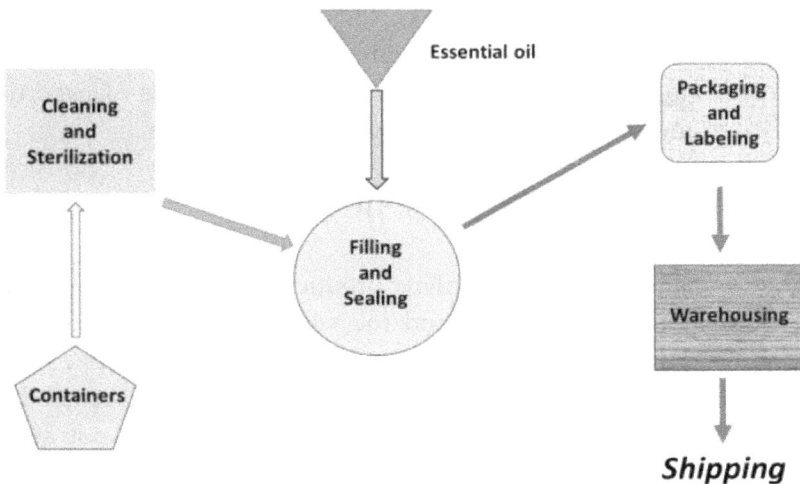

Figure 18.3 Schematic of the Young Living production process.

Capping of the bottles is automated, and this ensures that the caps with their security bands are air-tight to avoid any possible contamination and ingress of air or moisture. Likewise, labelling is automated, with each label indicating the product and lot number as well as a bar code to facilitate product identification in the warehouse and for filling orders. Thereafter, the filled, capped and labelled bottles are placed in partitioned boxes and transported to the warehouse.

Obviously, automated filling, labelling and capping systems are not used for small batches of oils and blends or when test or sample bottles are to be filled. In such cases, small-scale filling stations with customized filling systems and bottle cappers are used.

Some products are manufactured by subcontractors, e.g., bar soaps, dentifrices (toothpastes) and certain other Young Living specialty items. These products are manufactured in accordance with specific compositional and strict quality-control guidelines dictated by Young Living and are subjected to Young Living's QA/QC testing regimens. This approach has the great merit that Young Living can take advantage of the expertise and experience of other companies to produce premium quality products without the need to undertake the heavy investment in plant, equipment and personnel that is already available from select subcontractors. This approach is also adopted in the case of outside consultants, experts and advisers, and is very common with large corporations that rely upon high levels of expertise, knowledge and skill in their many and varied operations.

WAREHOUSING AND SHIPPING

Young Living produces a great many products with the inventory running into thousands of items, and the volumes of each product are prodigious. Further, thousands of items are ordered and shipped daily from Lehi, Utah to its members. As a result, there is a tremendous turn-over of items within warehousing, with goods going out at one end and newly-produced items replacing shipped products coming in the other end.

Several hundred call staff receive thousands of orders daily by telephone, email, fax, letter and the internet from Young Living members all over the world. Each order is assigned an individual bar code identifying the product, the customer and the shipping address. These orders are sent immediately to Warehousing where they are filled and loaded into individual cartons which are labeled and sent by a conveyor belt to Shipping. In Shipping, the order is scanned and checked for accuracy, packed, sealed and labeled before being packed into waiting carrier trucks for immediate dispatch within hours of the orders being received by Sales.

The scale of the operation, notably ordering, packing and shipping is enormous and incredibly efficient. Astonishingly, for such a large operation, consumer complaints are few and far between. Further, because of the efficient labelling and bar coding used throughout the filling, packaging and warehousing operations, errors in filling orders and shipping of products is almost unheard of.

Although the receipt of orders, digitizing, printing of packing sheets and labeling is a multi-faceted operation, the process is remarkably efficient and well-run. This is due to a sophisticated computer-controlled operation together with human inspection at critical points to ensure accurate filling of orders and to minimize any delays.

CONCLUSIONS

It should be obvious from this brief overview of the operations of a world-leader in essential oils that the *Seed to Seal* corporate logo of Young Living means just that. The Company grows its own plants from which it distills its spectrum of essential oils. All these plants are grown under environmentally-beneficent conditions using experienced personnel on company-owned farms throughout the world. Further, by growing their own plants, Young Living can guarantee that their products are wholly natural, 100% pure and are all obtained from known biocompatible sources.

As with harvesting, distillation operations are performed without delay, again assuring optimal yields and purity of the extracted essential oils. Because the corrosion-resistant and meticulously cleaned stills are operated by skilled and very experienced artisans, the distillation products are of the highest quality and greatest purity with minimal contamination by water or other distillation residues.

After the distillation products are collected, the extracted essential oils are subjected to extensive and very precise testing regimens to guarantee that only the highest purity products are released to members. The Seed to Seal and From the Ground Up philosophy and attention to every detail ensures the purity, quality and uniqueness of Young Living essential oils and their many products.

FINAL NOTE

It has been a remarkable experience to take a detailed look at the products and processes underlying the success of Young Living. Perhaps the greatest surprise to this author was the scale and extent of the Young Living organization and its processes and production as well as the diversity of membership within the Young Living "family". The total National and International membership now exceeds 6 million and is growing daily. This, in itself, is a very clear indication of both the quality of Young Living products and also that these products satisfy the needs and requirements of its members.

What was also a surprise was the extent of community support provided by Young Living and not to just to their members but to the general public when natural disasters occurred. Help was freely given by the company and its employees wherever and whenever it was needed.

This author was taken aback by the diversity of high-quality products supplied by Young Living and by the fact that new products, and improvements to existing products and devices, has been an ongoing company policy for decades. The company has never been content to sit back on its laurels as the premier essential oil company but continuously develops new and innovative products for its members. The scientific expertise and skill devoted to this approach is astonishing.

So, *Seed to Seal* is a wholly justified and highly commendable corporate logo for Young Living because everything the company does comes from plants grown in strict adherence to biodiversity and ecological conservation. High quality plants produce the highest quality essential oils and the processing, testing and evaluation of these oils ensures that every single product satisfies all quality, purity and

National and International standards. This book, entitled *Essential Oils from the Ground Up* is hopefully a fitting tribute to Gary Young, Young Living and all members of the Young Living Family. It has been my personal pleasure to share with readers what essential oils are, the incredible range of their properties and how they can markedly benefit and improve the quality of Life or users.

Thank you for taking the time to read this book and sharing in my pleasure at exploring the incredible world of essential oils.

APPENDIX A

Refractometry and Polarimetry

REFRACTOMETRY

It was indicated in Chapter 2 that seedlings are tested to ensure that they have optimal growth conditions and, should the need arise, growers can take appropriate measures to address any issues. Likewise, if growers can accurately gauge when plants have achieved their growth potential, they know that harvesting will yield the best possible plant material and, consequently, premium essential oils. Such measurements are made with a device known as a *refractometer* and the measurements are based on the optical effect known as refractometry.

Most people have seen the optical illusion of a pencil sticking out of water with the straight pencil appearing to be bent where it enters the water. This effect occurs because water has a different density to air, and light travels at a different speed in water than in air so that the pencil appears to be bent. Obviously, it is the light that bends, not the pencil. Clear liquids, glass, transparent crystals and many biological molecules also can "bend" a beam of light, the effect being known as *refraction*. Refraction is what gives diamonds and other gem stones their brilliance and sparkle, and it is the term used to denote the light-bending effect of fluids, Figure A.1

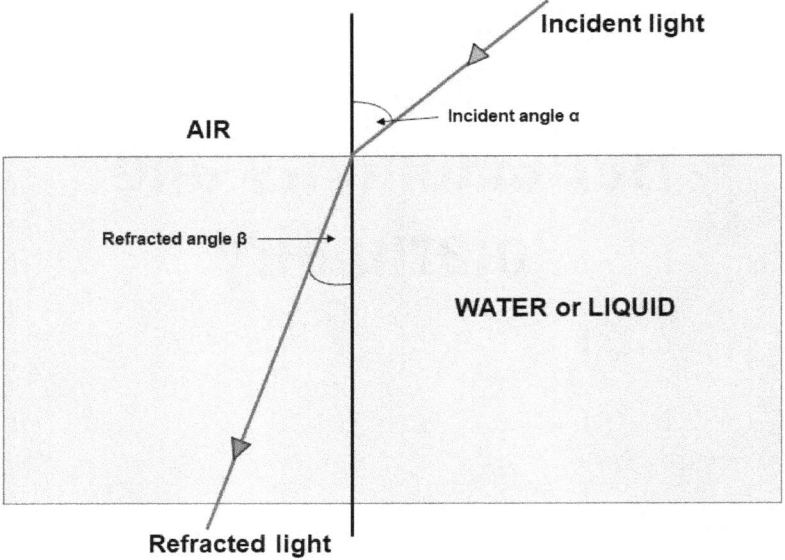

Figure A.1 Refraction of light caused by travel through a medium other than air.

Every transparent substance will bend or refract light at a different angle, depending on its specific gravity or density. In Figure A.1, the angle of the incident light (the angle at which the light strikes the surface) is denoted as α whereas the angle of refraction, i.e. the amount the light is bent, is denoted as β. This angle of refraction depends upon the second medium through which the light passes and can change with certain other conditions, notably temperature, light wavelength or frequency, magnetic effects and the concentration of the liquid medium. The way that materials and solutions will bend a light beam is known as the *index of refraction* or the *refractive index* for that substance at a specific temperature and is determined by the ratio of the angles α and β.

Some substances, for example, quartz crystal, will bend different frequencies (or wavelengths) of light at different angles with low frequency red light bending less than higher frequency blue light. As a result, when a beam of light is projected through a quartz crystal, it will be divided into bands of different frequencies and the refracted light is seen as a rainbow or spectrum of colors extending from red through violet.

The value of the refractive index of a solution is determined by means of an instrument known as a *spectrometer* and is used to detect and measure the elemental composition of complex molecules and mixtures. Back in the early 19th Century, a German physicist Joseph von Fraunhofer[116] observed what are now known as the Fraunhofer lines, a set of spectral lines in the optical spectrum of the Sun. Astronomers still use this principle and measure the refraction of a star's light as its signature spectrum to determine its elemental composition together with its distance from Earth and its speed.

In agriculture, measuring refraction provides information about the density of fluids, typically to measure soil moisture, irrigation water and plant fluids. This is because pure water at a specific temperature will bend or refract light at a specific angle, but any chemical dissolved in the water will change its density and thus change its refraction properties. Numerous biological substances when dissolved in water can increase the density of the solution, causing refraction of light as it passes through that solution. Measuring this change in the angle of refraction provides useful data on the density and chemical composition of the solution and its dissolved components (solutes).

In the case of plant sap, it is the sugars in the plant juice that are the primary cause of refraction. The second most abundant refractive substances in plant sap are mineral ions but because sap contains a higher proportion of sugars, which are larger in size compared to mineral ions, they have a greater effect on the solution's refractive index than minerals.

Brix is a technical term used to quantify and provide a numerical value for the amount that light is refracted on passing through a fluid

---

116 Joseph von Fraunhofer (1787–1826) was a direct ancestor of the author of this book.

and is named after Adolf Ferdinand Wenceslaus Brix[117]. In effect, the Brix value or number is a measure of the amounts of sugars and minerals dissolved in water or plant juices although many other chemicals that may be present can also contribute to the Brix reading.

A refractometer is the instrument used to obtain a Brix reading and is available in three basic types: optical, digital and laboratory. The first two types are handheld and simple to operate in the field so that growers can take regular and routine field measurements of plant sap density to check on their plants. The actual measuring procedure is relatively simple: sap is squeezed out of the plant onto the prism of the refractometer which is then pointed at a light source and then a reading is made. The image seen in the viewfinder of the instrument comprises a light and a dark field because part of the light beam passes through the thin film of plant sap while the rest bypasses the test specimen. The point at which the light and dark fields intersect is the Brix number, shown on a scale in the viewfinder.

Prior to the development of the refractometer, measuring the density of plant and grape juices was tedious but vital to the wine industry to assess the quality of wines. European winemakers could not predict which grape juices would make the best wine and the ability to judge quality ahead of actual wine making and bottling was of immense importance.

A major advance came much later with the work of Dr. Carey A. Reams (mentioned in Chapter 2) who showed that there were large differences in the mineral content of fruits and vegetables, depending on how and where they were grown. He went on to develop a Brix chart that covered most of the common fruits, vegetables and crops. Using Reams' Brix chart and refractometers, growers were able to adjust their growing methods and achieve higher quality food production. This approach to plant appraisal and evaluation is now central to growing botanicals for the essential oil industry.

---

117 Adolf Ferdinand Wenceslaus Brix (1798-1890), a 19th Century German chemist, mathematician and engineer was the first to measure the density of plant juices.

POLARIMETRY

Another nondestructive optical technique used to evaluate essential oils is polarimetry, a sensitive method of measuring the optical activity exhibited by inorganic and organic compounds. A compound is deemed to be optically active if linearly polarized light[118] is rotated when passing through it. This property of rotating polarized light is an important method of studying the structure of molecules and is widely used in quality control (QC), process control and research.

In particular, polarimetry is used to determine purity by measuring optical rotation by pharmaceutical products as well as a wide variety of essential oils. Polarimetry is also used to ensure product quality by measuring the concentration and purity of the many "sweet" compounds in sugar-based foods, cereals and syrups. The chemical industry uses optical rotation (polarimetry) to identify and characterize biopolymers, natural polymers and synthetic polymers. Interestingly, both the Food and Drug Administration (FDA) and the United States Pharmacopoeia provide polarimetric specifications for a great many compounds.

To understand the significance of polarimetry and why such measurements are made, it is necessary to introduce the subjects of *stereoisomerism* and *stereoisomers*. Two molecules are described as *stereoisomers* if they are made of the same atoms connected in the same sequence, but the atoms have different positions in space. In other words, the molecules have the same constitution, molecular formula and sequence of bonded atoms, but the three-dimensional orientations of their atoms in space are positioned differently. These molecules are known as *stereoisomers*. So, structural isomers have the same molecular formula but the bond connections or the ordering of these bonds are different for each molecule.

When two stereoisomers are reflections of each other, they are known as *enantiomers* or optical isomers because they are mirror images, in the same way that the left hand and right hand are mirror images of each other. However, these mirror images cannot be superimposed. This geometric property of some molecules and ions is known as *chi-*

---

118 *Linear polarization of light is when a beam of light* is confined to a single plane along the direction in which the light is travelling.

rality, the name coming from the Greek word for "hand" because the hand is a very familiar *chiral* object. So, a compound or system is *chiral* if it is distinguishable from its mirror image; that is, it cannot be superposed onto it. This is shown schematically in Figure A.2 for the biologically-important molecule, lactic acid.

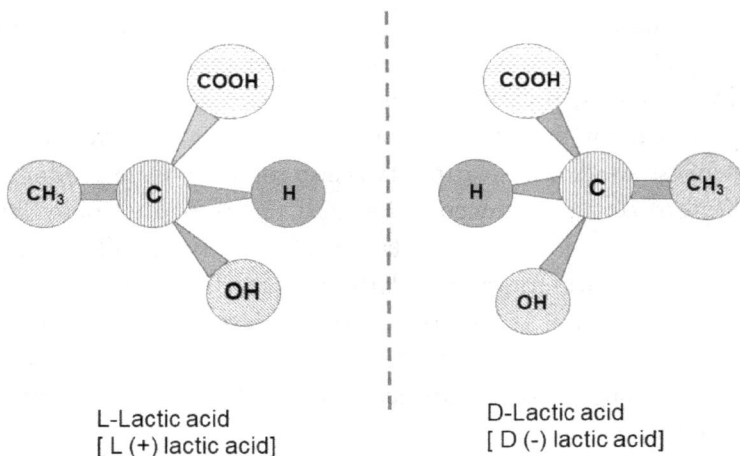

L-Lactic acid
[L (+) lactic acid]

D-Lactic acid
[D (-) lactic acid]

Figure A.2 L-lactic acid (left) and D-lactic acid (right) are non-superimposable mirror images of each other.

The two lactic acid isomers are known as L-lactate and D-lactate; L-lactate rotates light clockwise (+) and D-lactate rotates light counterclockwise (-). Because of this difference in light rotation, the molecule on the left is often known as L(+) lactate and the other as D(-) lactic acid. However, some chemists use the terms D and S to denote counter- and clockwise light rotation.

Chemically, two compounds that are enantiomers of each other have the same physical properties but are distinguished by two things. The first is the way they rotate polarized light and, secondly, how they interact with different optical isomers (enantiomers) of other compounds. The 2nd characteristic is highly significant because different enantiomers of a compound can have substantially different biological effects. This effect becomes even more complex with large molecules because there may be multiple chiral features in a given molecule or compound which, in turn, increases the number of geometric forms that are possible. Another characteristic of pure enantiomers is that they can only be separated with the use of a chiral agent, and such agents are often incorporated in chromatography columns (see Appendices C and D).

Because enantiomers often have different chemical reactions with other enantiomer substances and since many biological molecules are enantiomers, there sometimes can be a marked difference in the effects of two enantiomers on biological organisms. With drugs, for example, often only one of a drug's enantiomers may be responsible for the desired physiologic effects, while the other enantiomer is less active, inactive or sometimes can even cause adverse effects. One consequence of this effect is that a drug composed of only one enantiomer (a so-called *enantiopure* compound) can be developed to enhance its pharmacological efficacy and sometimes eliminate some side-effects.

Light sources, e.g. light bulbs, light-emitting diodes (LEDs) and the sun emit electromagnetic waves at the frequency of visible light. Their electric fields oscillate in all possible planes relative to their direction of propagation or beam. If light passed through a polarizer, only the part of the light that oscillates in the defined plane of the polarizer can pass through, that plane being called the plane of polarization; polarized light waves oscillate in parallel planes and are unidirectional. The plane of polarization is turned by optically active compounds and a *polarimeter* is a scientific instrument that is used to measure the angle of rotation of polarized light when passed through an optically active substance. Depending on the direction in which the light is rotated, the optically active enantiomer is referred to as *dextro*-rotatory or *levo*-rotatory, the latter meaning rotation to the left (counter-clockwise) and dextro-rotation means the light has been rotated to the right (clockwise). These optical rotational properties were mentioned above for lactic acid. The amount by which the light is rotated is known as the angle of rotation.

This principle of light rotation allows the ratio, purity, and the concentration of two enantiomers to be measured via polarimetry because the amount of optical rotation is proportional to the concentration of the optically active substances in solution. Polarimeters may therefore be applied to measuring the concentrations of enantiomer-pure samples. With a known concentration of a sample, polarimeters may also be used to determine the specific rotation when characterizing a new substance.

The net result of all this is that enantiomers may have identical chemical and physical properties except for their ability to rotate plane polarized light by equal amounts but in opposite directions and, for this reason, are often called optical isomers. A mixture of equal parts of an optically active isomer and its enantiomer is termed *racemic* and has zero net rotation of plane-polarized light because the positive rotation of each (L or +) form is exactly counteracted by the negative rotation of a (D or –) form. Natural substances such as pure essential oils are what are known as a racemic mixture, meaning they have equal amounts of left- and right-handed enantiomers of a chiral molecule. Consequently, polarimetric measurements of pure essential oils often exhibit minimal light rotation, which is an indication that the oil is a pure, natural substance. Interestingly, the first known racemic mixture was known as racemic acid, which Louis Pasteur identified as a mixture of the two enantiomeric isomers of tartaric acid.

The earliest polarimeters, dating back to the 1830s, were handheld and consisted of a tube with a polarizing element (the analyzer) at one end and another polarizer (the detector) at the other end. The optically active sample was placed in the tube which was held up to a light source, and the user had to manually turn the analyzer and judge the alignment when the least light was observed. The angle of rotation was then read to within one to two degrees from a simple scale fixed to the moving polarizer. Since those early days, there have been various refinements in polarimeters and both semi-automatic and fully automatic polarimeters are available and the results are now digitized. Despite these advances, the measuring principles remain the same, as is the usefulness of the data, although measurements are now made with greater speed and higher accuracy.

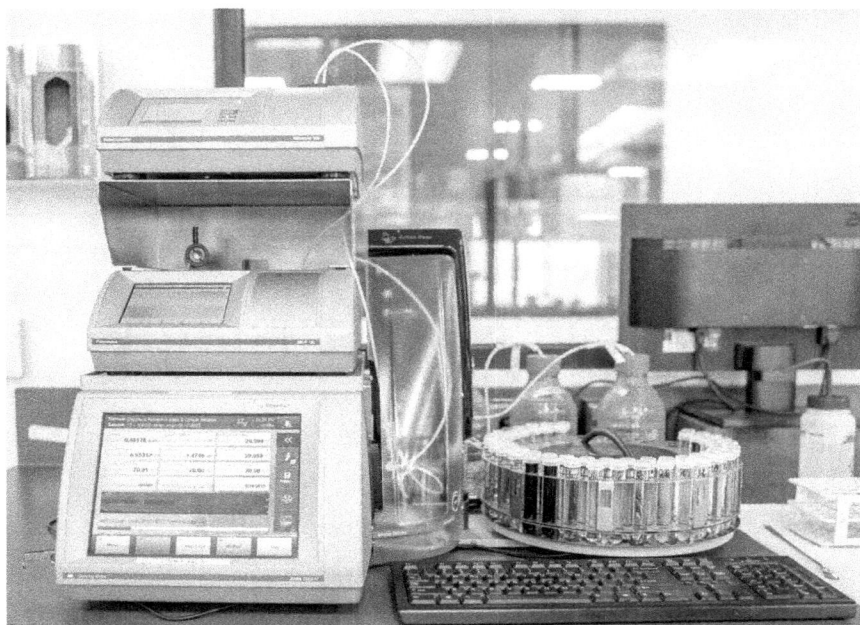

Figure A.3 Instrumentation used for Densitometry/Refractive Index/ Optical Rotation measurements [Courtesy of Young Living]

Interestingly, the very modern essential oil industry not only has ancient roots but also some of the oldest scientific technology is still routinely used to improve plants, ensure optimal growth and harvesting conditions, and accurately characterize the finished product. Although it is often said that there is nothing new under the sun, it can also be said that essential oils extracted back in ancient times bear little resemblance in terms of purity and biological efficacy to modern oils because of the continuous incorporation of modern science and testing methods in essential oil production.

APPENDIX B

Infrared Spectroscopy

Infrared spectroscopy is a chemical analysis method that is based on the interaction of infrared (IR) light with a molecule. However, before discussing IR spectroscopy, it might be useful to review some basic chemistry.

A chemical compound is simply a molecule made up of many atoms that are joined or bonded together. The characteristics of that compound are determined by the types of atoms making up the molecule and how those atoms are bonded together. Organic compounds (molecules) are mainly made up of carbon atoms bonded together, often in chains, whereas inorganic compounds are predominantly made up of the atoms of different elements.

When light is shone upon a compound, the energy in that light beam will be transferred to, and interact with, the atoms and their bonds in that molecule. The effect the light has on the molecule will depend on several factors but largely by the atoms and the interatomic bonds in the molecule, the wavelength (or frequency, which is the inverse of the wavelength) of the incident light and the light intensity. In general, the incident light causes the individual atoms to vibrate but also will make the atomic bonds vibrate and stretch. The actual effect will vary, in part, with the size or mass of the individual atoms, the bonds within the molecule as well as on whether the molecule contains groups of atoms, the latter being known as functional groups. In general, when irradiated with infrared light, stronger bonds between atoms will vibrate at a higher stretching frequency (wavenumber) than weaker bonds and lighter/smaller atoms will vibrate more than larger atoms.

IR spectroscopy is mainly used to determine the functional groups in organic (carbon-based) molecules. This is useful because the properties and reactions of chemical compounds depend upon the different functional groups within their molecules. The technique achieves this objective by measuring the absorption, emission or reflection of the incident IR radiation by a molecule. In other words, IR spectroscopy measures the vibrations of atoms and their bonds caused by the IR light impacting them. Then, based on the observed vibrations and the corresponding light absorption, this is used to determine the functional groups present in the molecule(s).

Individual atoms in a molecule are not identified by IR spectroscopy but the technique does indicate what kinds of bonds and functional groups are present in a molecule. Then, knowing what kinds of bonds and functional groups are present, the structure of the molecule (and often its identity) can be deduced.

The instrument that performs IR spectroscopy is known as an IR spectrophotometer and is shown schematically in Figure B.1.

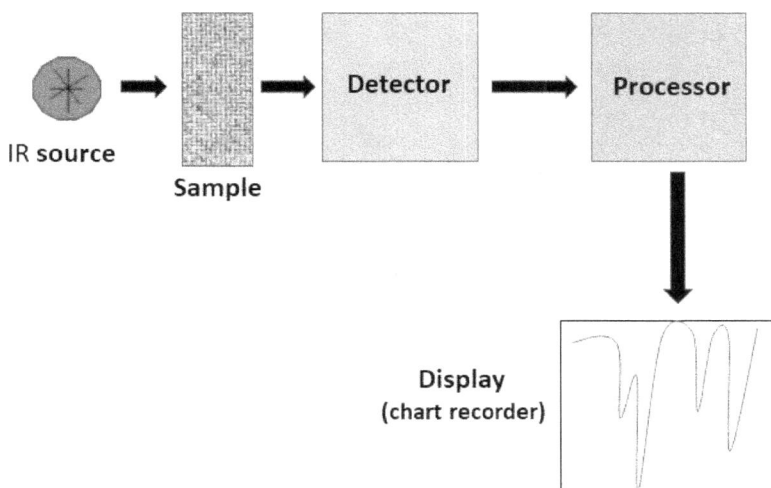

Figure B.1 Schematic diagram of a basic infrared spectrophotometer.

The basic principle of the instrument is that IR light within the wavelength range of 4000 to 600 cm^{-1} is focused on the sample, which can be a solid, a liquid or a gas. Light transmitted through the sample is measured by a detector and a processor is used to compare the light received by the detector with the incident beam of IR light. The processor measures the wavelengths of light that were absorbed by the sample and feeds this information to the display unit, usually a chart recorder. Thus, the IR spectrophotometer produces a plot of the measured IR light intensity versus the wavelength (or frequency) of the incident light and this plot or graph is known as an infrared spectrum.

Modern IR spectroscopy uses what is known as a two-beam absorption spectrophotometer, shown schematically in Figure B.2

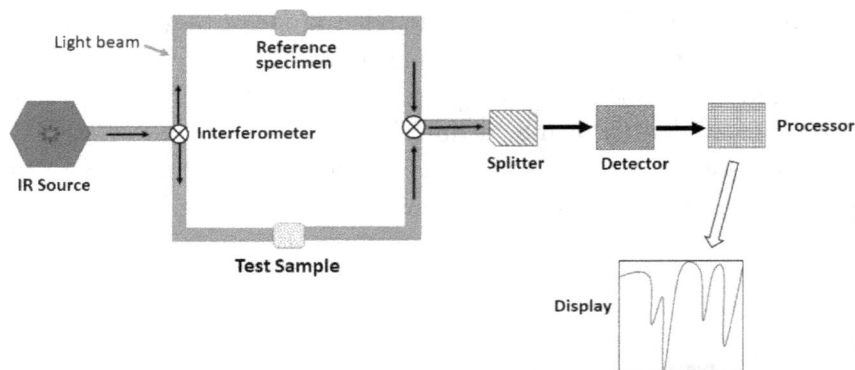

Figure B.2 Schematic diagram of a 2-beam IR spectrophotometer.

In a two-beam spectrophotometer, the infrared light is passed through an interferometer that splits it into two separate beams. One beam is passed through the test sample, the other is passed through a reference specimen. The two beams are then passed through a splitter that alternates between which of the two beams enters the detector. The detector compares the two beams and a printout or plot is obtained. This approach to obtaining an IR spectrum using both the test sample and a reference material has many advantages, including eliminating any problems within the detector, variations in beam intensity and largely eliminating errors due to the spectrophotometer itself.

Of course, advances in IR spectrophotometers are being made all the time and newer instruments have remarkably good electronics and computer software. An advance on the two-beam spectrophotometer and which is now almost an universal standard is known as Fourier Transform Infrared Spectroscopy or FTIR. In this approach, the IR light is guided through the sample and then through an interferometer while a moving mirror inside the apparatus alters the distribution of infrared light that passes through the interferometer. A detector measures the light output as a function of mirror position and produces an output known as an *interferogram*. The output from the detector is fed to a data processor which uses a mathematical method known as a Fourier transform to turn the raw data into an IR spectrum. The advantages of FTIR include increased accuracy, reduced background "noise" due to impurities, and greater operating speeds.

IR SPECTRA

Infrared spectroscopy produces what is known as an infrared spectrum. This is a plot of the measured infrared light intensity versus the wavelength (or frequency) of light. The peaks (actually they look like troughs) in the spectrum indicate which components in the molecule have absorbed infrared light.

It was discussed in Chapter 6, Figure 6.2, that a molecule's IR spectrum can be divided into the functional group region on the left and the "fingerprint region" on the right. The latter, extending roughly over the 1000-500 cm^{-1} wave number region, is always different or individual for each molecule. So, two different molecules may have similar functional group regions because they contain the same functional groups, but they will always have different fingerprint regions because of all the other atoms and bonds within the two molecules.

Identifying the functional groups over the wavenumber region of 4000-1500 cm^{-1} can be predicted based on detailed knowledge of the functional groups within a molecule using various theoretical calculations. They may also be identified by comparing the sample molecule's IR spectrum to the spectra for other molecules containing the same groupings. Of course, identifying the individual peaks in the fingerprint region on a theoretical basis is considerably more difficult, which is why the name is given to that region of the IR spectrum because, like human fingerprints, they are unique to the individual molecule (compound) under examination.

The fingerprint region is often used to distinguish between isomers. Isomers are compounds with the same formula but have a different arrangement of atoms in the molecule and different properties (see Appendix A). As an example, let's look at butanol, formerly known as butyl alcohol, and which has the atomic formula C_4H_9OH. Butanol can exist in different isomeric forms, but they all have the same chemical formula, i.e. they contain the same number of carbon and hydrogen atoms together with a hydroxyl (OH) group. These isomers have different structures and, consequently, their melting and boiling points, solubilities (miscibilities) in water and chemical properties are different.

The unmodified term *butanol* usually refers to the straight chain isomer with the alcohol functional group, (the hydroxyl group OH) at the terminal carbon, Figure B.3(a). This compound is known as *n*-butanol or 1-butanol. When the hydroxyl group is attached to a carbon atom along the chain, Figure B.3(b), the isomer is referred to as *sec*-butanol or 2-butanol. If the carbon chain is branched, Figure B.3(c), the compound is known as isobutanol or 2-methyl-1-propanol. Finally, the branched isomer with the alcohol grouping attached at the internal carbon, Figure B.3(d), is known as *tert*-butanol or 2-methyl-2-propanol.

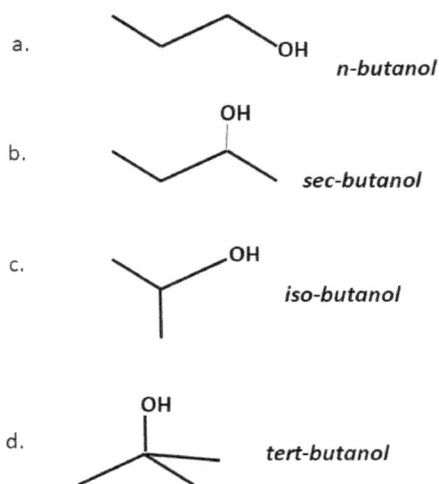

Figure B.3 Isomers of butanol

Distinguishing between the different isomers is usually a tedious and quite difficult analysis problem. However, whereas the isomers all have the same numbers of carbon and hydrogen atoms but different structures, the vibrations induced by infrared light will differ. Consequently, the "fingerprints" of the isomers will be different, and they can then be readily distinguished by IR spectroscopy.

It follows from this brief introduction that IR spectroscopy is a powerful tool for identifying compounds (molecules). However, it must be stated that when a mixture is being studied, identifying the individual compounds in that mixture can be difficult because each molecule will add its own absorption bands to the fingerprint region. The latter can then become quite "cluttered" and difficult to analyze even for skilled analytical chemists. Another problem that can arise is when a mixture containing a number of minor components is to be analyzed. In such cases, the characteristic spectra of the minor components are "lost" or indistinguishable in the fingerprint region because the latter is swamped by the major component in the mixture.

On the other hand, when a FTIR spectrophotometer is hooked to a chromatograph, it is then possible to identify each individual compound separated by the chromatography unit before IR spectroscopy is performed. This procedure is widely used in chemical analyses and in the pharmaceutical, petrochemical and polymer science industries as well as for essential oils and food analysis.

APPENDIX C

Chromatography

One of the mainstays of analytical chemistry is the methodology known as chromatography, a name derived from the words *chroma* (the Greek word for color) and *graphia* (meaning to write in Latin) or *graphein* (the Greek word for writing). Although this analytical technique is often mentioned on the wildly popular NCIS series, it actually is an old and well-established analytical technique. In fact, chromatography is a key weapon in the forensic scientist's arsenal in tackling drug analysis, detecting differences between organic and herbicide-treated foodstuffs and, of course, forensics.

Chromatography was first developed as a chemical analysis tool by the Russian scientist Mikhail Tsvet back in the 1910s which he used to separate plant pigments, notably chlorophyll and carotenes. Sadly, Tsvet's work was first published in Russian and largely ignored for decades but the technique gained resurgence after World War II. Since then, this analytical technique has made incredible strides with the advent of new technologies that have expanded the capabilities, accuracy and versatility of chromatography.

PRINCIPLES of CHROMATOGRAPHY

The underlying principle of chromatography is that it separates the components of a mixture by passing it through an inert medium in which the components move at different rates. The mixture can be a solution, a suspension or a vapor, the latter being known as gas chromatography. In other words, chromatography is a physical method of separation that distributes components to be separated between two phases, one being fixed (the stationary phase, usually contained in a column) whereas the other (the mobile phase) moves over or through the stationary medium in a definite direction. The eluate is the separated components of the mobile phase leaving the column.

There are many types of chromatography, each having a different name to indicate the actual method of operation. So, chemists may use a variety of chromatographic methods, such as liquid chromatography, thin layer chromatography, gas chromatography, ion-exchange chromatography and affinity chromatography to separate a mixture, but all techniques are based on the same basic principles. However, deciding which particular technique is used will be determined by many factors, including the nature of the sample (i.e., a liquid or a gas), the amount of material available for separation together with the skill and experience of the analytical chemist.

As a simple illustration of the basic principles of chromatography, look at Figure C.1. Two chemicals, reactants A and B, are mixed together and react to form compound C, the reaction product. The resulting mixture contains unreacted chemicals A and B together with the reaction product C. The mixture is then fed into a column that is filled with an inert material together with a carrier than moves the mixture down the column. Because the components A, B and C in the mixture have different size molecules, they will travel down the column at different rates. The actual transit time of the individual molecules through the column will be determined by the size of the molecules, the way they adhere to the column packing material, the flow rate of the carrier that moves them through the column and the type of material packing the column. This is known as the retention time of the eluate in the column.

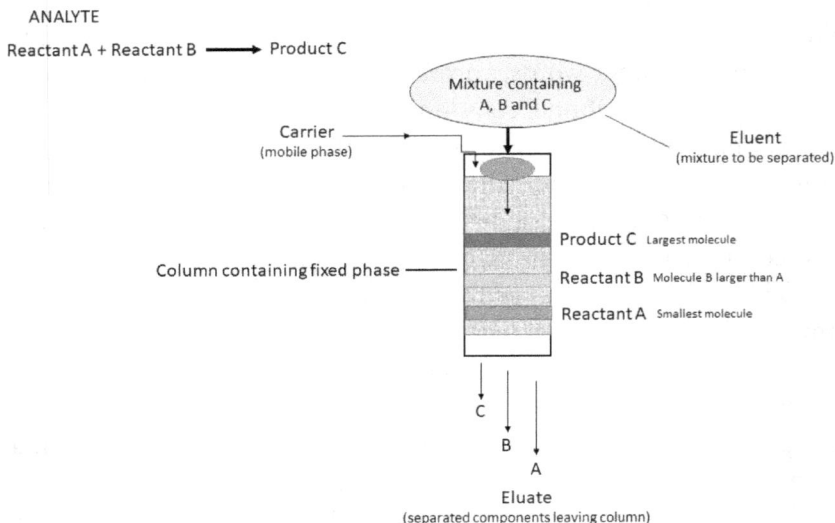

ANALYTE

Reactant A + Reactant B ⟶ Product C

Mixture containing A, B and C

Carrier
(mobile phase)

Eluent
(mixture to be separated)

Column containing fixed phase

Product C Largest molecule

Reactant B Molecule B larger than A

Reactant A Smallest molecule

C

B

A

Eluate
(separated components leaving column)

Figure C.1 Schematic diagram of a chromatography system.

The net result of a chromatographic separation is that the smallest molecule, reactant A, flows out of the column first, followed by reactant B, which has a larger molecule. Finally, the largest molecule, the reaction product C is delivered from the column. Thus, the three components in the starting mixture, the analyte, are separated and are collected individually, provided that the retention times of A, B and C through the column are different.

Obviously if the mixture contains a large number of components, then there will be an equally large number of bands that correspond to each individual component in the starting mixture. How the separated components are presented will depend on which particular chromatographic technique is used but, commonly, the separated mixture may be shown as a collection of individual bands, known as a chromatogram.

In the case of essential oils, which can be vaporized without breaking down or decomposing the oil, gas chromatography (GC) may be used to separate the individual components in the oil. Many factors are involved in specifying which column is used, notably the inert fixed phase as well as the dimensions of the chromatography column such as its diameter and length. Other factors include the carrier gas, the operating temperature, gas flow rates and other operating variables that are used to separate the components of a mixture. Again, efficient and effective chromatographic separation of multi-component mixtures requires experience, skill and a thorough understanding of the samples being studied.

Separating the mixture, however, is one thing whereas identifying each individual component requires an additional and usually completely different analytical technique. Various approaches are used for this task and these are discussed in Appendix E.

APPENDIX D

Mass Spectrometry

Mass spectrometry (MS for short) is an analytical technique that breaks down and ionizes chemical species and characterizes (identifies) them based on their mass-to-charge ratio.

In essence and very simplified, the sample, which may be a solid, liquid, or gas, is ionized in the mass spectrometer by bombarding it with electrons. This bombardment causes some of the sample's molecules to break into charged fragments or ions. These ions then are separated based on their mass-to-charge ratio by accelerating them in an electric or magnetic field so that they are turned or deflected. Ions of the same mass-to-charge ratio undergo the same amount of deflection and they are detected by a device known as an electron multiplier. The mass spectrometer will produce a chart or spectrum showing the relative abundance of detected ions as a function of the mass-to-charge ratio. The atoms or molecules in the sample can be identified by correlating known masses to the identified ions or through a characteristic fragmentation pattern from known reference samples.

THE MASS SPECTROMETER

A mass spectrometer comprises three components, shown schematically in Figure D.1.

1. The Ionization Chamber or source: typically, a high energy beam of electrons ionizes the sample material fed into the instrument, usually to form cations through the loss of an electron, e.g. a sodium atom (Na) when ionized loses an electron e⁻ to form a sodium cation (Na⁺):

$$Na \rightarrow Na^+ + e^-$$

In this example, the Na⁺ ion has single charge and its mass will be that of the sodium atom.

In operation, gases and volatile liquid samples are injected into the ion source from a reservoir whereas solids and non-volatile liquids may be introduced directly into the ion source chamber. In action, different ionization methods have been developed for different types of samples to be analyzed by mass spectrometry. This causes some of the sample's molecules to break into charged fragments and the generated ions are then accelerated and focused into a beam.

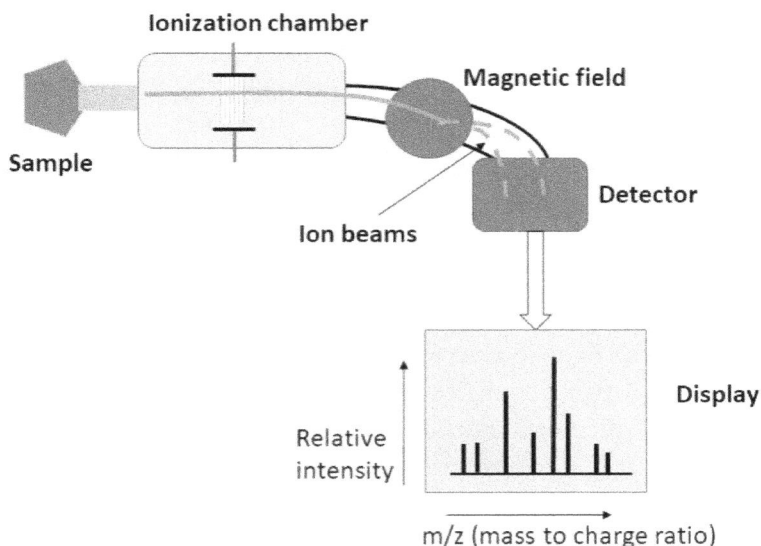

Figure D.1 Schematic diagram of a mass spectrometer.

2. The Mass Analyzer: The beam of ionized material is fed into the mass analyzer and manipulated by external magnetic fields (or

sometimes electric fields) to separate the ions based on their mass and charge. What happens is that the magnetic field, which is positioned perpendicular to the ion beam, accelerates the ions in the beam which is deflected in an arc that has a radius inversely proportional to the mass of each ion. For a magnetic field of given strength, lighter ions are deflected more than heavier ions. Consequently, by varying the strength of the magnetic field, ions of different mass can be focused progressively on a detector fixed at the end of the curved tube.

3. The Detector: measures the separated ions in the ion beams and the results are displayed on a chart.

In other words, what the mass spectrometer does is break the sample down into its component parts and then measures the masses of the separate components to produce a mass spectrum. The latter is a plot or graph of the ion signal governed by the mass-to-charge ratio of each component in the mixture. The resultant spectra are used to determine the elemental or isotopic signature of a sample, namely the masses of particles and the parent molecules. This information is used to determine the chemical structures and identities of the molecules. It should be noted that the results of mass spectrometry may depend heavily on sample preparation, the instrumentation used and how the analysis was performed.

To correctly evaluate the MS spectrum, pure and unambiguous standards must be used to calibrate the system so that the resulting spectrum can be interpreted accurately. Nowadays, large libraries of mass spectra are available to simplify the identification of a sample and to quantify the component parts of a mixture. In particular, mass spectrometry can be used to measure molecular mass, molecular structure and sample purity but each of these determinations requires a different experimental procedure. Further, accurate identification of the components of a sample requires proper and carefully controlled data collection while interpretation of the spectrum must be based on known standards to ensure accuracy.

The important point to remember about mass spectrometry is that it is a highly effective and sensitive analytical tool, even where there is only a small quantity of sample is available for analysis. On the other hand, analyzing mixtures is often difficult and special techniques are used for this task, as discussed in Appendix E.

APPENDIX E

Characterizing Mixtures

Chromatography can separate mixtures into their individual components but does not identify them, and other analytical techniques are required to characterize and identify the individual molecules. Infrared spectroscopy and mass spectrometry are both incredibly accurate in characterizing a particular molecule but identifying that molecule, however, is far more difficult. Although abstruse theoretical and mathematical calculations can perform this task, the usual approach is to use known standards against which the sample's IR and MS spectra are compared so that the unknown molecule can be identified. Many instruments now have extensive spectra/spectrogram libraries within their hardware and software so that these comparisons and analyses can be performed automatically, rapidly and with great accuracy. Problems arise, however, when a mixture containing two or more components must be analyzed. Neither IR or MS can readily distinguish between a mixture of different molecules, and a different approach must be adopted.

Chromatography, Appendix C, is primarily a technique that separates mixtures. However, unless special instrumentation (especially the detectors) are used, chromatography cannot distinguish between different but similar molecules that take the same amount of time to travel through the column and, consequently, two or more molecules can elute at the same time. Therefore, a secondary analytical technique is required to identify each molecule as it is eluted from the chromatography column.

Infrared spectroscopy produces spectra (see Appendix B) that are characteristic of the molecule in the sample. However, when several molecules are present, distinguishing between the mixture's components can be very difficult. If the mixture is separated, for example by chromatography, then each component can be identified separately and in turn as it elutes from the chromatography column.

Likewise, mass spectrometry (Appendix D) normally requires a very pure sample and when there are impurities present or the sample contains several different molecules, then it is possible that two different molecules in a sample can have a similar pattern of ionized fragments. The result is that the mass spectrometer cannot distinguish between the molecules in the sample. However, if the components in the mixture are separated by, for example, chromatography, then each component in the mixture can be individually identified.

Consequently, analytical chemists combine two or more analytical techniques to identify and characterize a mixture. Thus, while it is not possible to accurately identify a particular molecule in a mixture by gas chromatography, infrared spectroscopy or mass spectrometry when used alone, combining two or more techniques does make this possible. A common approach to this is the combination of gas chromatography (GC) and mass spectrometry (MS), a methodology known as GC-MS. Viewers of popular TV series such as NCIS are probably quite familiar with the many references to the use of GC-MS in analyzing trace matter found at crime scenes.

A GC-MS instrument produces a mass spectrum, which is a plot or graph of the ion signal as a function of the mass-to-charge ratio of each component in the mixture. The GC part of the instrument (the gas chromatograph) separates the mixture and each separated component is fed in turn to the MS part of the instrument (the mass spectrometer). The resultant spectra of the separated components in the mixture then are used to determine the elemental or isotopic *signature* of a sample, namely the masses of particles and the parent molecules. This information will help an experienced chemist to characterize the chemical structures and identities of the molecules present in the original mixture. A schematic diagram of a GC-MS instrument is shown in Figure E.1.

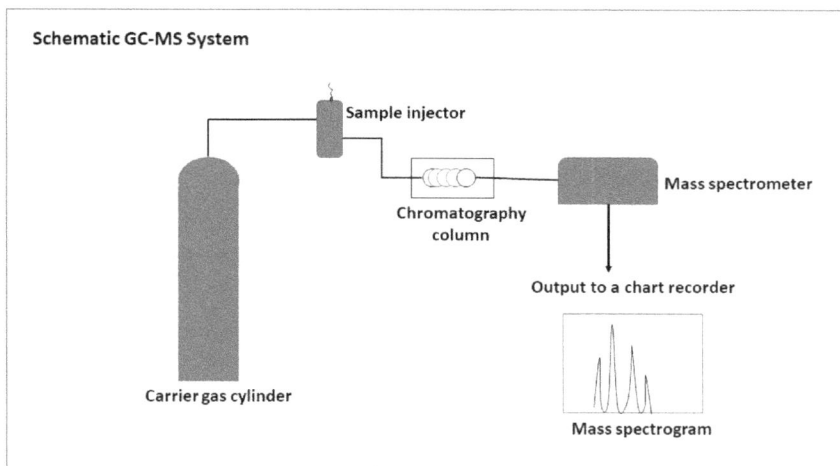

Figure E.1 Schematic GC-MS analysis system.

The GC-MS combination reduces the possibility of error because it is highly unlikely that two different molecules will behave the same way in <u>both</u> a gas chromatograph <u>and</u> a mass spectrometer. Therefore, the mass spectrum that appears at a characteristic retention time in a GC-MS analysis (i.e. characterizing each eluate from the gas chromatograph in turn) ensures that there is far greater certainty that the sample analyte under investigation is identified.

As mentioned in Appendix D, pure and unequivocal standards are used to calibrate the system for accurate evaluation of MS spectra. Fortunately, large libraries of mass spectra exist that make identification and quantification more-or-less straightforward with GC-MS. Nevertheless, the results can also depend heavily on sample preparation, the instrument used and how the analysis was performed.

GC-MS is very useful for analyzing mixtures and, particularly, distinguishing between synthetic and natural products, e.g. essential oils. The following GC-MS chromatograms for synthetic and 100% natural wintergreen oils show this very clearly.

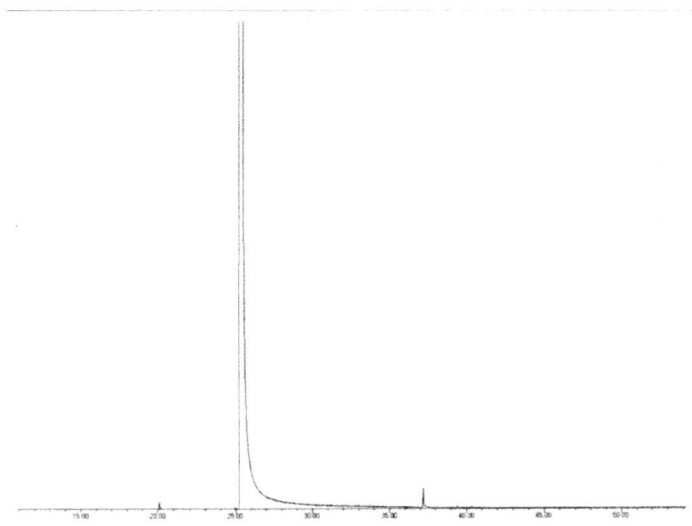

Figure E.2 GC-MS chromatogram of synthetic wintergreen oil [Courtesy of Young Living].

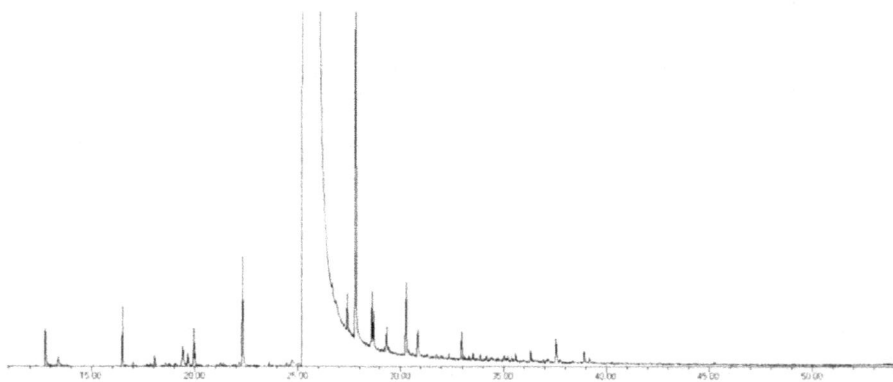

Figure E.3 GC-MS chromatogram of genuine (100% natural) wintergreen oil [Courtesy of Young Living].

The chromatogram in Figure E.2 shows that the synthetic wintergreen oil contains methyl salicylate as the primary ingredient together with a small amount of ethyl salicylate (the smaller band at the higher m/z ratio to the far right of the major lines). In contrast, the chromatogram of the 100% natural wintergreen oil, Figure E.3, shows the characteristic lines for methyl salicylate together with a number of bands for the other naturally occurring components present in the oil. Further, the natural oil contains minimal amounts of ethyl salicylate, as shown by the missing line for the compound which would have been there at a higher m/z ratio. Obviously, GC-MS can be used to unequivocally distinguish between synthetic and wholly natural essential oils, an analysis routinely performed by Young Living chemists on virtually all commercial products that are available on the wholesale and retail markets.

GC-MS can clearly distinguish between nominally the same essential oils available from different manufacturers. This is because there will always be differences in the relative amounts of the principal and minor components in the oils so that the chromatograms will be characteristic for each individual oil. Basically, they will be highly individual "fingerprints" for the oils. As a corollary, GC-MS will also readily distinguish or indicate commercial products that have been adulterated or contain diluents. In other words, GC-MS will clearly show when the purported essential oil is neither 100% pure nor a 100% natural product.

APPENDIX F

Bacteria and Microbiological Testing

Essential oils are extracted from plants by distillation, a process that involves heat and, because they are oils, they are water-free. Consequently, as mentioned in Chapter 6, they should be free from bacterial contamination. Despite these factors and the fact that microbial contamination is highly unlikely, microbiological testing is still routinely performed. As a responsible manufacturer of essential oils, Young Living always quarantines its extraction products for a minimum of 5 days after distillation and performs microbial tests before any other chemical or physical analysis is performed to ensure that their products are bacteria- and virus-free. For this reason, it might be useful to briefly review bacteria and microbiological testing for the sake of completeness.

Bacteria are microscopic living organisms or *microbes* that are found everywhere but which require water or an aqueous environment to exist. They can be dangerous and cause infections (i.e., these are the pathogenic or "bad" bacteria) or they are beneficial to the body and its biochemical processes (i.e., the "good" bacteria). Good bacteria include those present in probiotics and yoghurt as well as those involved in fermentation processes such as wine making, digestion in animals, decomposition of animals and plant remains and sewage disposal. In contrast, pathogenic bacteria cause severe and often fatal diseases in humans, animals and plants. In fact, the first bacterial disease ever discovered was anthrax, caused by the bacterium *Bacillus anthracis,* and which was identified in cattle and sheep in 1876.

Bacteria occur singly or in chains and have different shapes. Rod bacteria, as the name implies, are microbial species with a rod shape whereas a coccus (plural: cocci) is a spherical or ovoid-shaped bacterium. A cluster of bacteria with the appearance of a bunch of grapes is labelled "*staphylococci*" whereas chains of clustered bacteria are called "*streptococci*". Many cocci are pathogenic, causing a variety of diseases, including "strep. throat", pneumonia, meningitis, gonorrhea and rheumatic fever, to name but a few.

Finally, a word about bacterial nomenclature. The name of the *genus*[119] or family of bacteria is italicized and followed by *spp.,* e.g. *Bifidobacterium spp.* refers to the genus of Bifidobacteria which reside in the healthy human digestive tract. It is common in microbiology to shorten the name of a particular genus of bacteria to a single capital letter, usually italicized, with a second word indicating the particular species. For example, with the bacterium *Escherichia coli*, commonly referred to as *E. coli, Escherichia* is the genus and *coli* the species.

CLASSIFYING BACTERIA

Bacteria are classified into two main groups based on the structure of their cell walls. The classification system and method of identifying bacteria by staining was developed by the Danish physician and bacteriologist, Hans C. J. Gram. Because of differences in the cell walls of the bacteria, a *Gram-positive* bacterium acquires a purple/blue color in Gram's staining method whereas a *Gram-negative* bacterium takes on a pink/red color.

For humans, animals and plants, the vast majority (about 90-95%) of Gram-negative bacteria are pathogens and cause disease whereas most Gram-positive bacteria are non-pathogenic and usually

---

119 *Genus* is defined as the usual major subdivision of a family consisting of more than one species, e.g. the Latin term for modern man is Homo sapiens, where the word *Homo* refers to genus and *sapiens* refers to species.

beneficial to the body. They are also widely used in other applications. The subject of Gram-positive and Gram-negative bacteria and their effect on the body is discussed in greater detail below because of their importance regarding probiotics.

PLANT BACTERIA

Most plant pathogenic bacteria belong to the genera (or generic names) listed in alphabetical order in Table F.1 below. These pathogenic bacteria cause many different symptoms in plants, including galls, overgrowths, wilts, leaf spots, specks, blights and soft rots, as well as scabs and cankers.

> *Acidovorax*
> *Agrobacterium*
> *Burkholderia*
> *Clavibacter*
> *Erwinia*
> *Pantoea*
> *Pectobacterium*
> *Phytoplasma*
> *Pseudomonas*
> *Ralstonia*
> *Spiroplasma*
> *Streptomyces*
> *Xanthomonas*
> *Xylell*

Table F.1 Pathogenic plant bacteria.

Whereas it is often assumed that plant and human bacterial diseases are distinct and cannot cross over from plant to the grower or gardener, this actually is not the case, and although human infection from plants is very rare, but it does occur. The primary pathogen of concern is the common Gram-negative, rod-shaped bacterium *Pseudomonas aeruginosa,* which is a bacterium pathogenic to plants, animals and humans. *P. aeruginosa* is known for its ubiquity as well as for its multidrug resistance, notably its antibiotic resistance and its association with serious illnesses such various sepsis syndromes and hospital-acquired infections such as ventilator-associated pneumonia. This bacterium is opportunistic in that serious infection often occurs during existing diseases or conditions, notably traumatic burns and cystic fibrosis. *P. aeruginosa* infections in humans can invade nearly any tissue in the human body and the symptoms vary widely, and can include urinary tract infections (UTIs), gastrointestinal (GI) infections, dermatitis and even systemic illnesses. Although *P. aeruginosa* infections are rare and are becoming increasingly antibiotic resistant, they only become serious when the immune system is weakened or compromised. In fact, the infection rate of *P. aeruginosa* is very low (about 0.4%) even in severely ill, hospitalized patients. In other words, it is highly unlikely that an otherwise healthy person will ever develop an infection even if there are open wounds that come in contact with infected plant tissues.

Plants may also develop viral infections but, in common with plant bacteria, it is very rare for humans to become infected by plant viruses. For the vast majority of people with normal-functioning immune systems (i.e., non-immunocompromised individuals), the risk of human infection from plants is highly improbable. Nevertheless, although quarantining of essential oil distillates and microbiological testing is only an extra precaution, such procedures ensure the safety of Young Living essential oils and their oil blends.

GRAM-NEGATIVE BACTERIA

The staining behavior of Gram-negative bacteria and the major cause of their pathogenicity is the structure of the cell membrane. When the cell wall breaks down, a bacterial toxin known as an *endotoxin* within the body of a bacterium is released. If the endotoxin enters the bloodstream and so may reach any part of the body, it can cause a pathological effect such as a toxic reaction. The symptoms of a toxic reaction are that the sufferer develops a high temperature (known as a *pyrogenic* effect), accelerated respiration and low blood pressure, and this sometimes may lead to fatal endotoxic shock.

Although millions of Gram-negative bacteria are present in the gut, endotoxin released by these bacteria is detoxified and eliminated by the liver in healthy individuals. However, if the level of endotoxin increases beyond what can be detoxified by the liver and starts spreading through the body, the immune system releases an inflammatory substance and causes the body temperature to rise and fight the infection. When the levels of endotoxin in the blood go above what can be controlled by the immune system, endotoxic shock can occur. Before this happens, antibiotics should be administered to deal with the infection. However, when an antibiotic is administered to tackle Gram-negative bacteria, it is essential that the patient complete the prescribed course of antibiotics in order that they have completed their task and eliminated the infection, but also to prevent the Gram-negative bacteria from developing resistance to these prescribed antibiotics.

GRAM-POSITIVE BACTERIA

The most important Gram-positive bacteria are bacilli (rod-shaped microorganisms) and cocci (spherical or ovoid in shape). Certain Gram-positive bacteria are pathogenic, but the majority are beneficial to the human body, i.e. they are the "good" bacteria, and are often mentioned in regard to probiotics.

Lactobacilli are Gram-positive, rod-shaped "good" bacteria that are found as single cells or chains in the *flora* (i.e. collections of bacterial species) of the mouth and the vagina. Certain *Lactobacillus* species are involved in the production of yogurt, sour cream and buttermilk and many bacteria within this species are the principal components of probiotics formulations.

Bifidobacteria spp. are Gram-positive anaerobic bacteria that are one of the major microbial species in the gastrointestinal (G.I.) tract, vagina and mouths of mammals. *Bifidobacterium* species are also important probiotics and are used in the food industry for their many beneficial health effects. These benefits include regulation of bacterial balance within the intestines and inhibition of pathogens that colonize and/or infect the gut mucosa.[120] *Bifidobacterium spp.* also discourage the growth of Gram-negative pathogens in infants.

---

120 Gomes AMP, Malcata FX. *Bifidobacterium* spp. and *Lactobacillus acidophilus*: biological, biochemical, technological and therapeutical properties relevant for use as probiotics. Trends in Food Science & Technology (1999) 10 (4-5) 139-157.

Pathogenic ("Bad") Gram-positive bacteria

Streptococci are spherical bacteria that occur as chains with some streptococcal species being aerobic and others are anaerobic (these terms are explained below). Although there are harmless streptococcal species involved in the production of yogurt, buttermilk and cheese, others are decidedly pathogenic. These include *Streptococcus pneumoniae*, the cause of secondary bacterial pneumonias, and *Streptococcus pyogenes*, the causative agent of "strep throat".

Staphylococci occur in clusters and are normally present on the skin and in mucous membranes, but certain species are involved in skin pathologies such as boils, abscesses and carbuncles. *Staphylococcus aureus* is involved in such serious conditions as food poisoning, toxic shock syndrome, pneumonia, staphylococcal meningitis as well as MRSA (methicillin-resistant *Staph. Aureus*) infections.

AEROBIC and ANAEROBIC BACTERIA

Bacteria are also classified into two groups - aerobic and anaerobic - based on their requirement of oxygen. Anaerobic bacteria (anaerobes) can survive without oxygen whereas aerobic bacteria (aerobes) grow and multiply only in the presence of oxygen.

There are three types of *anaerobic* bacteria. These are *obligate anaerobes* which cannot survive in the presence of oxygen, *aerotolerant* anaerobes which do not use oxygen for growth but can tolerate its presence, and *facultative* anaerobes, which can grow without oxygen but can use oxygen if it is present. Some anaerobic bacteria are pathogenic and can cause sinus infections, colds, fevers, ear infections and sexually transmitted diseases like syphilis, gonorrhea and chlamydia. A common *facultative* anaerobe is *E. coli* (*Escherichia Coli*) which is present in the intestinal tract of human beings, mammals and birds but which can cause acute respiratory problems, diarrhea and urinary tract infections. *E. coli* outbreaks often occur with contaminated foodstuffs.

Staphylococcus is a genus of facultative anaerobe that are found on the mucous membranes and human skin, and the aggressive species, *Staphylococcus aureus*, was mentioned above. Anaerobic bacterial infections can be difficult to treat and often require extended antibiotic treatment or specialized topical applications for recalcitrant infections such as those involved in deep-seated problems with the skin and bone fractures such as osteomyelitis.

Microorganisms that require oxygen for cellular respiration, i.e., they need oxygen to survive, grow and reproduce are known as *obligate aerobic* bacteria although, as mentioned above, facultative bacteria (such as *E. coli* and *Staphylococcus spp.*) can behave both aerobically and anaerobically, depending on the prevailing conditions. There are also *microaerophilic* bacteria which require oxygen for their survival but only at a very low concentration. An example of a microaerophilic bacterium is *Helicobacter pylori (H. pylori)*, which is present in patients that suffer from chronic gastritis and gastric ulcers although over 80% of individuals infected with the bacterium are asymptomatic (i.e. have no symptoms). Interestingly, *H. pylori* may play an important role in the natural functioning of the GI system. The major roles of aerobic bacteria within the body are in the recycling of nutrients and decomposing waste products within the GI system.

ANTIBIOTICS

There are vast numbers of pathogenic bacteria which cause disease although the body is programmed to destroy invasive bacteria through the immune system. If the immune system of the patient is compromised and cannot deactivate bacterial infections, these pathogens customarily are dealt with by antimicrobial agents such as antibiotics. The latter enhance or augment the immune system's ability to deal with pathogens either by killing bacteria (*bactericidal* action) or slowing their growth by inhibiting their multiplication (*bacteriostatic* action).

The first antibiotic was penicillin, discovered in 1928 by Sir Alexander Fleming, and it ushered in the antibiotic era. Medicine changed forever in the early 1950's, when large scale production of penicillin became possible. The term "antibiotic" originally was applied only to antimicrobials derived from living organisms such as molds and yeasts. In contrast, "chemotherapeutic agents" are purely synthetic in origin although they have bacteriostatic or bactericidal activity against pathogenic microorganisms. Nowadays, all antimicrobials are known as antibiotics, including naturally-derived, semi-synthetic and wholly synthetic therapeutics and individual antibiotics vary widely in their effectiveness against different species of bacteria. Conventional antibiotics, however, are not effective in nonbacterial infections such as those caused by viruses or fungi.

Antibiotics typically are classified by target specificity. Narrow-spectrum antibiotics are used to treat particular types of microorganisms, e.g. specifically Gram-negative or Gram-positive bacteria, whereas broad-spectrum antibiotics can treat a wider range of bacteria. The effectiveness of an individual antibiotic varies with the type of infection, the infection site and its ability to reach that site through the blood supply to that site. Antibiotic efficacy also depends upon the ability of the bacteria to resist or inactivate the administered antibiotic. Whereas antibiotics are considered to be relatively harmless to the host, hence their use in treating infections, they often have an adverse effect on indigenous bacteria, particularly those within the gut. This is where probiotics, and their beneficial effects on the GI tract, come in.

During the latter part of the 20th century and now into the 21st Century, the clinical effectiveness of antibiotics has been decreasing, in some cases alarmingly so, e.g. MRSA or methicillin-resistant *Staph. aureus* infections. There are various causes of this problem, notably overuse and/or inappropriate administration of antibiotics as well as mutations within many bacterial species resulting in antimicrobial resistance. Consequently, many bacterial species are resistant to all antibiotics and the overall prevalence of antibiotic resistance is rising, with some 60% of *nosocomial* (hospital-acquired) infections now being antibiotic-resistant. This problem has in part stimulated study of essential oils to treat bacterial infections.

MICROBIOLOGICAL TESTING

Accurate and definitive microorganism identification and pathogen detection is essential for correct disease diagnosis, treatment of an infection with appropriate antibiotics and forensic investigation of outbreaks of diseases caused by microbial infections. Bacterial identification also is used in a wide variety of applications, including criminal investigations, forensics, evaluating bio-terrorism threats and environmental studies.

Identifying and Classifying Bacteria

The known characteristics of different bacteria have been compiled in a multi-volume reference work called *Bergey's Manual of Systematic Bacteriology*. The first edition of this important work was written[121] back in 1923 but has been continuously revised and updated since then. The identification schemes of Bergey's Manual are based on morphology (e.g., coccus, bacillus, etc.), staining (Gram-positive or negative), cell wall composition (e.g., presence or absence of peptidoglycan[122]), oxygen requirements (e.g., aerobic or anaerobic) and biochemical tests, such as whether the bacteria can metabolize or ferment sugars.

Traditionally, bacteria were identified by what is known as *phenotyping*, that is, identifying the bacterium by such characteristics as its morphology (i.e., the shape of the bacteria), biochemical properties, how it develops or proliferates when cultured and Gram staining. However, because some bacterial strains may have unique biochemical characteristics that differ from patterns that have been used as characteristic of known species for decades, more advanced techniques such as DNA testing have been increasingly employed over the last 15-20 years.

The most fundamental technique for classifying bacteria is the previously mentioned Gram stain, which is called a differential stain because it differentiates among bacteria and can be used to distinguish them based on differences in their cell wall. In the Gram staining methodology, bacteria are first stained with crystal violet dye and then treated with an iodine-potassium iodide mixture to fix the stain inside the cell. Then the bacteria are rinsed with a decolorizing agent like alcohol, followed by counterstaining with safranin, a light red dye.

---

121 David Hendricks Bergey, University of Pennsylvania.

122 *Peptidoglycans* are a molecular network of certain chemicals (carbohydrates) known as disaccharides, the latter being the water-soluble sugars formed when two monosaccharides are chemically joined; three common examples are sucrose, lactose, and maltose.

The cell walls of Gram-positive bacteria (e.g., *Staphylococcus aureus* or *S. aureus*) have more peptidoglycans than those of Gram-negative bacteria. As a result, Gram-positive bacteria retain the original violet dye and cannot be counterstained.

The cell walls of Gram-negative bacteria (e.g., *Escherichia coli* or *E. coli*) are much thinner and have an outer layer both chemically and structurally different to Gram-positive bacterial walls. This outer layer is disrupted by the alcohol wash and, as a result, the first dye washes out and the cell can then take up the second dye or *counterstain*. The net result is that Gram-positive bacteria will stain violet whereas Gram-negative bacteria stain pink. Gram staining is most effective with young, growing populations of bacteria, and there can be inconsistent results with older bacterial populations, typically those that are maintained in laboratories.

In addition to the Gram stain, bacteriologists/microbiologists may use other stains to distinguish particular microbial species such as *Mycobacterium tuberculosis* (the cause of tuberculosis) and to detect the presence of spores and flagella. There are also various laboratory tests available to identify disease-causing organisms, an important consideration when physicians must determine which antibiotic or other medication to use to treat an infection.

Another important bacterial identification technique is based on the principles of *antigenicity* which is the ability of the immune system to stimulate the formation of antibodies. Solutions of antibodies against specific bacteria (*antisera*) are commercially available and these are used to identify unknown organisms. The procedure involves mixing the unknown bacteria in a drop of saline with antisera that has been raised against a known species of bacteria. If the antisera cause the unknown bacteria to clump together or *agglutinate*, then the test positively identifies the bacteria as identical to that against which the antisera was raised. The test can also be used to distinguish between strains of bacteria, i.e. those that are slightly different but belonging to the same species.

There are, of course, many other test methods used to identify bacteria, but these are beyond the scope of this book. In bacterial testing of essential oils, however, precise identification of any possible microbial contaminants is less important that determining whether or not any such contaminants are actually present.

Test procedures

When an essential oil is tested for the presence of bacteria or other microbial species, sample drops are placed on a nutrient medium or gel contained in a glass or plastic container known as a Petri dish. After the Petri dish is "plated", it is placed in an incubator so that any bacteria present can grow.

In microbiology, the term *colony forming unit* or CFU is often used and refers to the number of colonies (clumps of bacteria) growing on the surface of the gel. Microbial growth is measured by the increase in the bacterial population, either by measuring the rise in cell numbers or the increase in overall mass. The basic method of evaluating bacterial growth is by cell or bacterial colony counting with various methods being available for this task. These approaches include visual observation, flow and turbidity measurements, biomass determinations and even nutrient uptake. The results are commonly expressed as an MIT value, which is the time that microorganisms are exposed to the test media and then are visually inspected for viable microorganisms.

If no growth of bacteria or other microorganisms occurs within a specified time for the Petri dish "plated" with the essential oil, then the sample material is declared to be free of microbes and then can be evaluated for its other properties, see Chapter 6.

APPENDIX G

Common Food Allergens

The American Academy of Allergy, Asthma, and Immunology (AAAAI) has stated that 20% of Americans suffer from allergies or hypersensitivity reactions, which are defined as the abnormal reaction of the body's immune system to an allergen. The symptoms can range from mild responses such as hives to severe reactions, even to death. Mild and possibly moderate allergic reactions are often relieved by topical and systemic applications/ingestion of anti-histamines but in severe cases, more aggressive approaches and even hospitalization may be necessary.

Clearly when about one in five (20%) Americans suffers from one or more allergies throughout the year, eliminating dietary sources of allergens is a simple and logical approach to ease suffering. The commonest food allergens are noted here in the frequency order of occurrence.

NUTS

Peanut allergies constitute over 3.3 million allergy cases in the U.S., and this prevalence has virtually eliminated packages of peanuts being distributed as snacks on airlines and most schools strive to exclude any and all nut exposure for children. The reason for this apparent over-reaction to peanut exposure is because, of all food allergens, reactions to peanuts are typically the most severe, causing the highest rates of anaphylactic[123] shock compared to other types of allergies. It should be noted that peanuts, peanut butter and peanut oil are present in many foods such as stews and chili, and in beauty products and moisturizers. Cross-contamination by peanut oil can also be a problem with many processed and fried foods, and even in restaurant foods.

SHELLFISH

One of the more common food allergies is late-onset shellfish allergy which affects over 2% of American adults. Sufferers must avoid clams, crabmeat, lobster, mussels, oysters and shrimp as well as dietary supplements manufactured from shellfish (e.g. glucosamine), certain pet foods as well as potential cross-contamination in restaurants.

EGGS

Egg allergies are more common in children (afflicting about 1%) than adults, and sensitivity to egg whites is more customary than to yolks; about 20% of pediatric sufferers find that sensitivity to this allergen can carry over into adulthood. Interestingly, breast-fed infants can have an allergic reaction to egg proteins in breast milk if the mother consumes eggs. Unfortunately for sufferers, eggs are present in a great many food-stuffs, notably mayonnaise, meringue, salad dressings, custards, puddings, pastas, baked goods, breaded foods and processed meats. Egg proteins are also present in influenza and yellow fever vaccines, both of which are made in eggs. On the other hand, the very important **Measles-Mumps-Rubella (MMR) vaccines** are generally safe for children with egg allergy despite eggs being involved in their manufacture.

SOY

Soy, like egg protein, is a more common allergen for children than adults but, again unfortunately, soybeans and soy sauce are present

---

123 *Anaphylaxis* is a rapid onset and very serious allergic reaction that can lead to death. Typical symptoms include one or more of the following: hives (itchy rash), swelling of the throat or tongue, shortness of breath, vomiting, lightheadedness and hypotension (low blood pressure).

(obviously) in oriental foods, many packaged foods, baby formula and a variety of hair and skin products.

MILK

Cow's milk may be the most common food allergen because of its ubiquity. Some 80% of U.S. children can suffer from exposure to dairy products, and this sensitivity, like that with pediatric egg and soy allergies, can carry over into adulthood. Milk allergy is an immune response to the proteins in milk and can occur even with lactose-free products. It is different from *lactose intolerance*, which the term given to the body's inability to digest milk sugars.

WHEAT

Wheat (gluten) allergy is not the same as the autoimmune disorder celiac disease but can result in significant health challenges, including anaphylaxis in sufferers exposed to both wheat and physical exertion. Unfortunately for sufferers, wheat is found in so many things, including (obviously) bread and baked goods, breakfast cereals, deli meats, most brewed beverages (beers) and soy sauce, some cosmetics and hand creams, moisturizing lotions and shampoos. In this context, it is interesting that Young Living produces numerous products fabricated from the ancient grain Einkorn which has a naturally low gluten content.

SALT and SUGAR

Although salt and sugar are generally not allergens, they are endemic to modern society and the modern (21st Century) diet, and both can have devastating effects on health. Prepared (packaged) foodstuffs as well as restaurant foods are laden with salt while sugar is present in almost everything including bread, soft drinks, cereals and even "healthy" foods like milk and yoghurt. Most people are aware that a high salt diet will raise blood pressure and sugary foods can lead to acne, tooth decay and obesity. What is less known is that sugar intake is related to decreases in HDL (the "good" cholesterol), new-onset depression, respiratory disease, hypertension, liver disease, periodontal disease and even squamous cell carcinoma. Even worse news for people with a "sweet tooth" is that there is mounting evidence that artificial sweeteners like saccharine, sucralose and aspartame can damage the microbiome[124] of the gut. Restricting salt and sugar intake can markedly improve health.

---

124 The collection of microbes that live in and on the human body is known as the *microbiota* whereas the term *microbiome* refers to the complete set of genes within these microbes.

APPENDIX H

Topical Use of Essential Oils for Common Problems

[®: Young Living proprietary oil blend; *: Tea tree oil]

The following comments indicate the pure essential oils and essential oil blends used by many individuals as first aid treatments and are for educational purposes only; they have not been evaluated by the Federal Food and Drug Administration (FDA) and are not meant to be used to diagnose, treat, cure or prevent any disease.

Problem	Conventional Approach	Essential Oils Remedy
Acne	Antibiotics, pre-scription drugs	Melaleuca*, Lavender
Blisters	Puncture, drain, apply antibiotic cream or petroleum jelly	Lavender
Bruises	Apply ice, elevate	Helichrysum, Geranium, Fennel, PanAway®

Burns	Antibiotic creams, hydrocortisone, sunlight	Lavender, Geranium, Melaleuca
Colds/sinus/ allergies	Antihistamines, decongestants, analgesics	Peppermint, Breathe Again®
Corns	Salicylic acid ointment	Clove
Cuts, skin scrapes, shallow wounds	Antiseptics, antibiotic creams	Lavender, Helichrysum, Basil, Melaleuca.
Dandruff	Anti-dandruff, conditioner-based shampoo	Rosemary, Wintergreen
Depression, anxiety	Antidepressants	Lemon, Frankincense, Peace & Calming®, Stress Away®
Fever	Analgesics	Peppermint
Fungal infections	Prescription antifungal agents, OTC medications	Melaleuca, Cinnamon, Clove, Thyme, Oregano
Headaches/ pain	Analgesics	Peppermint, Stress away®
Hives (urticaria)	Antihistamine	Melaleuca, Peppermint
Indigestion, upset stomach, nausea	Antacids, Tums®, Pepto-Bismol®	Peppermint, Ginger, Lavender
Inflammation and swelling	OTC anti-inflammatory medication, Calendula ointment	Frankincense, Melaleuca, Eucalyptus, PanAway®
Insect bites, stings, rashes	Antihistamines, calamine, hydrocortisone	Basil, Melaleuca, Melrose, Copaiba, Helichrysum, Roman Chamomile, Purification®
Insect repellant	Chemical sprays, Off®	Citronella, Patchouli, Lavender, Purification®

Insomnia, sleep problems	Unisom®, melatonin, prescription drugs	Lavender, Peace & Calming®
Muscle ache, joint pain	Analgesics, embrocations	Cool Azul®, PanAway®, Deep Relief®
Muscle cramps	Gentle massage, ice and analgesic ointment.	Lemongrass + peppermint, Marjoram, PanAway®
Pain (localized)	Analgesics, Analgesic ointment	Lavender, Eucalyptus, PanAway®, Deep Relief®, Cool Azul®
Parasites	Anti-parasitic and anti-inflammatory drugs	Oregano, Thyme, Fennel, DiGize®
Poison Ivy and Poison Oak	Clean, Calamine lotion, Hydrocortisone ointment/cream	Lavender, Eucalyptus, Cypress, Geranium, Rose, Myrrh, Melaleuca, Joy®
Rashes	Calendula cream,	Geranium, Rose, Lavender
Ringworm	OTC antifungal cream, lotion or powder	Melaleuca, Oregano
Scars	Mederma®, prescription scar creams	Lavender, Frankincense, Helichrysum
Skin cleaning and purifying	Soap, Cetaphil®, Proactiv®, Eucerin®	Basil, Thieves Waterless Hand Purifier®, Thieves Cleansing Soap®, Young Living bath gels.
Sore throat	Cough drops, throat spray	Thieves lozenges®
Stretch marks	Mederma Stretch Marks Therapy®	Helichrysum, Sage, Rose, Lavender, Neroli, Patchouli
Toothache	Clove oil	Clove, Purification®

Warts	OTC wart ointment	Frankincense, Melaleuca, Oregano, Clove, Thieves®
Wrinkles	Cosmetics	Frankincense

INDEX

ABOUT THE AUTHOR

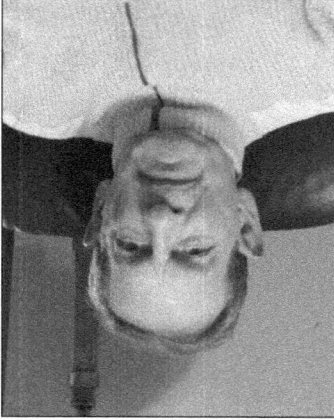

Photograph by Susan A. Lake

Dr J. Anthony von Fraunhofer is an Internationally-recognized expert in biomaterials science and the properties and behavior of materials used in dentistry and medicine as well as industry. He has lectured and presented seminars in many countries and has written over 450 scientific papers, 19 books, and contributed chapters to 15 monographs. In addition to his ongoing research activities and peer-review of submissions to professional journals, he has broadened his fields of interest to include the properties and characteristics of essential oils.